Modern Biotechnology

Methods & Advances

Dr. MORTAGY   RASHED

Table Contents:

Introduction

Biotechnology is technology based on biology, especially when used in agriculture, food science, and medicine. The UN Convention on Biological Diversity has come up with one of many definitions of biotechnology: "Biotechnology means any technological application that uses biological systems, living organisms, or derivatives thereof, to make or modify products or processes for specific use."

Modern biotechnology is often associated with the use of genetically altered microorganisms such as E. coli or yeast for the production of substances like insulin or antibiotics. It can also refer to transgenic animals or transgenic plants. Genetically altered mammalian cells, such as Chinese Hamster Ovary (CHO) cells, are also widely used to manufacture pharmaceuticals. Another promising new biotechnology application is the development of plant-made pharmaceuticals.

Biotechnology is also commonly associated with landmark breakthroughs in new medical therapies to treat diabetes, Hepatitis B, Hepatitis C, Cancers, Arthritis, Hemophilia, Bone Fractures, Multiple Sclerosis, Cardiovascular as well as molecular diagnostic devices than can be used to define the patient population. Herceptin is the first drug approved for use with a matching diagnostic test and is used to treat breast cancer in women whose cancer cells express the protein HER2.

We see tremendous progress in the research of gene makes us feel puzzled, every day we discover new, but that the great successes achieved by the science in the field of communicating quickly dropped the line between what we can do today, and we appreciate him for the moment, between the present and Mammal to do tomorrow. for example, procreation find the issues that worry biological yesterday no longer hold their attention, or perhaps become a priority in their present research, as there is great difference between the means used by the science of birth control and minimize reproduction in the middle of this century, for example, between the sophisticated technology that enables us to control the genetic characteristics of embryos in this day.

Eight great achievements in the field of biology and genetic engineering is no longer limited impact on the manufacture of genetically or a formation genetic characteristic of human beings, but it has gone for that to include the feelings and self-aspects.

What you that the issues of pregnancy and childbearing is no longer subject to traditional vaccination, because modern techniques keeping eggs as example, transport and planting in the wombs of women Chance had facilitated us many options.

we opened the door to alternatives were unthinkable until recently one has been able rights in the near future to create copies thanks to technical uniformity quite sophisticated.

The fungal and congenital diseases and disabilities, it can eliminate or mitigate the impact of years at least, through controlling gene for the disease as genetic or impairments resulting from the flaw affects the reform of the same gene defect before the birth of the fetus would eliminate those diseases and disabilities that science unsophisticated and technology are now pose on the scene in recent decades, the problems of moral concern and deserves reflection , For as much as to the outcome of our knowledge and increase our ability to control things and allow us new options always raise new issues revolve around what is right and what is wrong. The criteria identify right and wrong it turned stem from the actual needs of Rights does not necessarily from the traditional sources. In an era of science explosive in this era of advanced technology, has become a touchstone of the complex morality approaching slowly from the reality of the situation that already exists rather than ideals paradox. Indeed, it would not have to change our ethical and turn it not for the era we live variable is already causing significant shift speed.

Recently and still live revolutions in various areas of science impending rights achievements in the fields of corn, electronics, and the conquest of space, but the biology is a scientific revolution in the present day. Through this study on the topic of biotechnology will focus on the two important issues, Methods and Advances, which raise the interest of scientists and researchers in this moment.

MORTAGY RASHED

CHAPTER 1

Genetic Engineering

Genetic engineering is a part of the biological revolution in modern evolution passed through four primary stages: 1) Phase biological phones. 2) Phase molecular biology. 3) The stage of genetic engineering. 4) A vital called cloning.

The scientists realized the importance of genetics discovery of the nature or inherited gene, to change a lot of appearances and hereditary diseases, in 1953 discovered the nature of this gene at the hands of (James Watson) and (Craig Francis),

Where it became apparent to them that (DNA) molecule consisted of two series complementary of sugar and phosphate and nitrogenous bases, and takes these two tapes form snails.

There are certain points converge each All the other tape carries full information necessary to control the building of proteins required to guide the vital operations of the total interaction leads in the end to the organism. When the cell divided and separated two series attracts each of the chemical elements of nitrogenous bases is completed, and give us a new structure of peaceful Cyclones double. In this way, the cell maintains the new genetic codes found in the mother cell. It was this discovery significant role in founding the science of genetic engineering and the emergence of the reestablishment of (DNA) or control genes, arriving after the so-called therapeutic vital.

The term genetic engineering is often thought to be rather emotive

Or even trivial, yet it is probably the label that most people would

Recognize. However, there are several other terms that can be used to describe the technology, including gene manipulation, gene cloning, recombinant DNA technology, genetic modification, and the new genetics.

There are also legal definitions used in administering regulatory

Mechanisms in countries where genetic engineering is practiced

Although there are many diverse and complex, techniques involved,

The basic principles of genetic manipulation are reasonably

Simple. The premise on which the technology was based on genetic

Information encoded by DNA and arranged in the form of genes.

A resource that can be manipulated on various ways to achieve certain Goals in both pure and applied science and medicine.

There are many areas in which genetic manipulation is of value, including the

Following:

_ Basic research on gene structure and function

_ Production of useful proteins by novel methods

_ Generation of transgenic plants and animals

_ Medical diagnosis and treatment

_ Genome analysis by DNA sequencing

In later chapters, we will look at some of the ways in which genetic

Manipulation has contributed to these areas.

The mainstay of genetic manipulation is the ability to isolate a

Single DNA sequence from the genome.

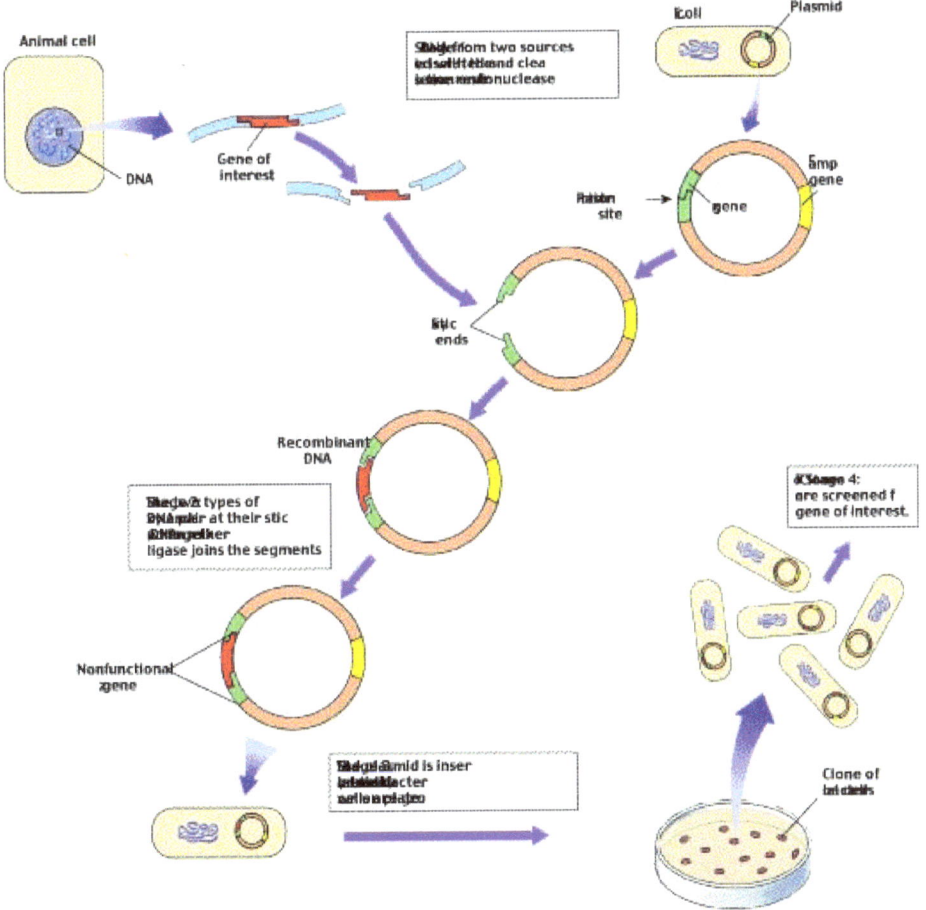

Stages in a genetic engineering experiment. In stage 1, DNA containing the gene of interest (in this case, from an animal cell) and DNA from a plasmid are cleaved with the same restriction endonuclease. The genes amp and lacZ′ are contained within the plasmid and used for screening a clone (step 4). In step 2, the two cleaved sources of DNA are mixed together and pair at their sticky ends. In step 3, a recombinant DNA is inserted into a bacterial cell, which reproduces and forms clones. In Stage 4, the bacterial clones will be screened for the gene of interest.

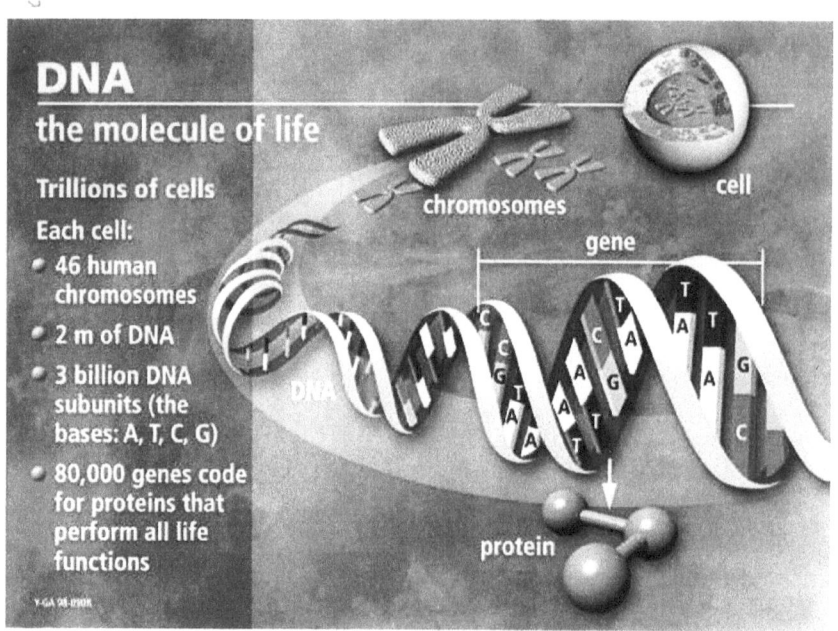

Elucidation of the structure of DNA caused a lot of excitement in the scientific community for two principal reasons. First, the structure suggests an obvious way in which the molecule can be duplicated, or replicated, since each base can specify its complementary base by hydrogen bonding. Thus, each strand can serve as a template for the synthesis of a complementary strand. Second, the structure suggests that the sequence of nucleotide pairs in DNA is dictating the sequence of amino acids in a protein encoded by a gene. In other words, some genetic code may comprise information in DNA as a sequence of nucleotide pairs, which can be translated into the different language of amino acid sequence in protein.

CHAPTER 2

Gene Technology

The future of human genetic engineering has made strides and made harvests scientifically unique promise to remove worries and disease, millions of people and opened new horizons in the way of treatment and diagnosis, possibly change the face of the map health early in the next century, especially in the field of diagnosis and treatment of genetic disease and cancer and the diagnosis of viral diseases and genetic testing. (GENE THERAPY) Diseases result of the technology revolution gene (GENE TECHNOLOGY) and the accurate knowledge of the installation of genes in the chromosomes (colored objects) which carry genetic characteristics of the human person and include every molecule in his body, whether color of eyes or hair color length or various other attributes in addition to the findings of modern science to specific enzyme (RESTRICTION ENZYMES) can be explored genes responsible for the human qualities of each individual and whether to remove pathogens, as well as a gene transfer systems (GENE TRANSFER SYSTEM), which can transport genes to the desired rights. Genes have two: 1) the production of materials for the continuation of the life of cells. 2) production of materials needed body such as insulin and various hormones and correct the error, which happens to these genes lead to the correct track, and therefore the possibility of cure hereditary diseases, it is clear that gene therapy in its simplest form is to introduce genes and functional (FUNCTIONAL GENE) to the cells of the patient to replace the genes infected either because of a genetic disease or unearned. Through DNA analysis which holds rights within the body can map gene everyone has been identified about 40 thousand genes hereditary while the goal is access to knowledge between 75-100 genes, through the huge project funded by the United States and cost three billion dollars and employ hundred plant and will be attended by several countries in the world.

The gene map is a way designed to identify qualities rights and good vision allowing know the real picture and full respect for all human health in terms of growth and development diagnosis and subsequent treatment future in the light of genetics and the discovery of individuals who are willing to certain diseases and work in every way to prevent morbidity and preventive methods on the environment in some cases because the disease is not as a result of genetic factors, but the result of the interaction of genetic factors and environment as exposure to radiation, pesticides and some medicines, cigarette smoke and other factors motivating.

The past years have witnessed dozens of attempts to cure gene For example , During the 1994 (the inauguration) is the first real beginning and promising to develop what was known with a suicide gene therapy for cancer, and scientists expect that the great revolution happening in the future in dealing with cancer, after they achieved very good results at the level of principle with particular types skin cancer as Ironically, scientists are strong indications that the possibility of success with cancer of the gastrointestinal tract, throat and esophagus tumors and diseases of the contract deployed sporadically in the human body.

In a nutshell the idea of gene therapy to introduce similar time bomb in tumor cells where explode once Docking cancer cell lead to the crash of cancerous cells or genes to cancer cells make toxic materials sorted and thus the crash itself .

Gene technology is the term given to a range of activities concerned with understanding the expression of genes, taking advantage of natural genetic variation, modifying genes and transferring genes to new hosts.

Gene technology sits within the broader area of biotechnology – the use of living things to make or change products. Humans have been using biotechnology for centuries in activities ranging from plant and animal breeding through to brewing and baking.

As our understanding of how living things function, grow and reproduce increases, modern biotechnology creates new opportunities for food and fiber production.

Modern biotechnology includes the discovery of genes (genomics) understanding how genes function and interact (functional genomics) development of natural DNA markers to select more plants that are efficient and animals and genetic modification or genetic engineering.

Gene technology is rapidly improving.

The polymerase chain reaction (PCR) is a laboratory technique that can produce many copies of a gene or segments of a gene, which makes studying the gene much easier. A particular segment of deoxyribonucleic acid (DNA), such as a particular gene, can be copied (amplified) in the laboratory. Starting with one DNA molecule, at the end of 30 doublings (only a few hours later) about a billion copies are produced.

Various methods may be used to determine (probe) changes in genes. A gene probe can be used to locate a specific part of a gene (a segment of the gene's DNA) or the whole gene in a particular chromosome. Probes can be used to find normal or mutated segments of DNA. A DNA segment that has been cloned or copied becomes a labeled probe when a radioactive atom or fluorescent dye is added to it. The probe will seek out its mirror-image segment of DNA and bind to it. The labeled probe can then be detected by sophisticated microscopic and photographic techniques. With gene probes, a number of disorders can be diagnosed before and after birth. In the future, gene probes will probably be used to test people for many major genetic disorders simultaneously.

An oligonucleotide is a chain of bases (nucleotides). Sometimes these chains are missing or have duplicate segments of DNA. An oligonucleotide array is used to identify deleted or duplicated segments of DNA in specific chromosomes. In an oligonucleotide array, DNA from a person is compared to a reference genotype using many oligonucleotide probes. Like some gene probes, a fluorescent dye is added to the oligonucleotide probes. If a part is missing, the probes detect a decreased amount of the fluorescent dye. If a part is duplicated or tripled, the probes detect an increased amount of the fluorescent dye. These probes can be used to test the entire genotype.

Microchips are powerful new tools that can be used to identify DNA mutations, pieces of ribonucleic acid (RNA), or proteins. A single chip can test for millions of different DNA changes by using only one sample.

Newer technologies can detect even smaller parts of genes and DNA by breaking the entire genotype into small segments and then analyzing the DNA sequence of some or all of the segments. A powerful computer then analyzes the results. Single variations in bases may be identified as well as very short segments of bases. Some of these variations can help doctors diagnose genetic disorders. Some of the newer technologies called next-generation sequencing are so sensitive that doctors can detect DNA from the fetus in a sample of blood drawn from the mother and analyze it to determine whether the fetus has Down syndrome. However, the error rates of such testing are still being determined.

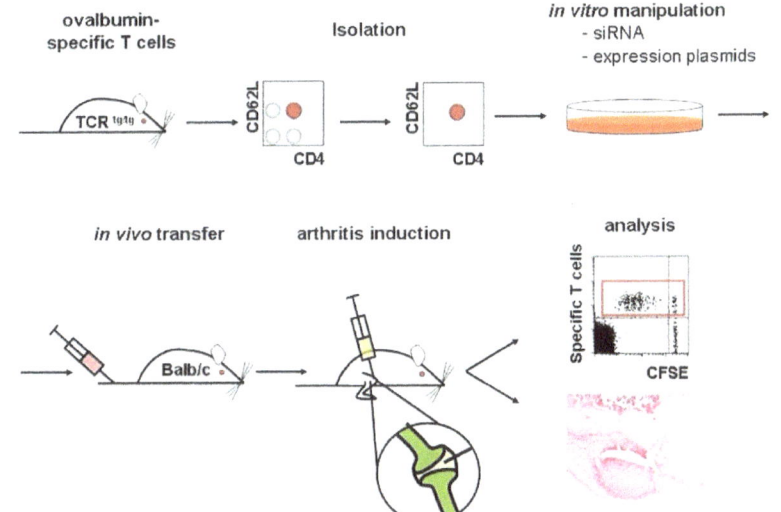

ovalbumin-
specific T cells
Isolation
in vitro manipulation
- siRNA
- expression plasmids

in vivo transfer
arthritis induction
analysis

Experimental system for the functional gene analysis in T cells in in vivo disease models. T cells derived from TCR-tg/tg mice can be transfected in vitro to overexpress or knockdown a previously identified target gene. The modified T cells populations can be transferred into non-transgenic cells and the effect of the gene modification on the antigen-specific immune reaction and disease development can directly be analysed.

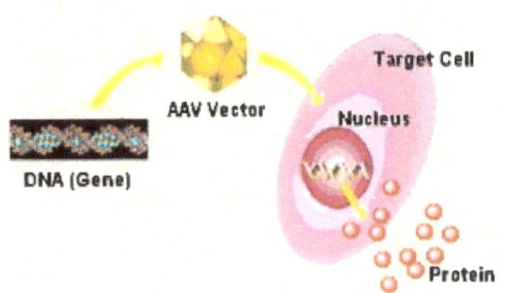

DNA (Gene)

AAV Vector

Target Cell

Nucleus

Protein

Sure enough, the treatment produced lasting improvement in the animals. After the gene therapy, blood-clotting times dropped from more than an hour's time to 15 to 20 minutes. Normal clotting time in healthy animals is about six minutes. It took about two months for the genes to maximize expression of the missing protein. The researchers were encouraged to find that expression levels remained stable for more than a year after the one-time treatment. Moreover, no side effects or limiting immune responses occurred as a result of treatment.

CHAPTER 3

Prostate Cancer

A method for the treatment of prostate cancer surgery, radiotherapy or hormonal.

.Surgical treatment is the extermination of the prostate island or radiotherapy is the best way rooted in the early stages of treatment in the case of the spread of the disease to parts of the body in the form of both high schools in the system or lymph glands or other body parts are treatment the use of hormones, and using this method will control the disease for a long time, but if there colonies of cancer cells are not sensitive to Hormones, leading to the spread of the disease again. The pace of genetic therapy is a significant step in the direction of overcoming carcinomas, which afflict many prostates. Where, a team of scientists to find a new vaccine was prepared in the methods of genetic engineering are expected to have an active influence in helping patients with this type of cancer who have not responded to conventional treatment methods.

This method relies on the amendment recipes cancerous cells from secondary tumors by infusing new vaccine to turn cancerous cells from the elements urges object to the composition of objects existing anti-cancer by leading to the break the growth of secondary cancers and places its inception in prostate.

During testing researchers have found a gene activated responses immune system has been encouraged cells to kill cancer cells and then planted inside the skin of rats suffering from prostate cancer and later became mice able to get rid of the cancerous cells and when they are approved this treatment system on humans, it will save millions of patients who suffer or died of prostate cancer every year.

Recent advances in immunology, tumor biology, and genomics have paved the way for the development of gene-based therapy. With the task of sequencing and identifying all human genes well under way, the first tentative steps toward clinical trials using gene-based treatment of urologic cancers, including those of the bladder, renal cell, and prostate, have begun.

Gene therapy is a new form of treatment in which a functioning gene is inserted into a cell to correct a specific genetic defect or to target a particular molecular pathway that can alter disease at its most fundamental level.

The prostate is an especially suitable target for gene therapy, since it is expendable after the reproductive years and is easily accessible through a Trans rectal, Trans peritoneal, or transurethral approach. Furthermore, using the regulatory sequences of prostate-specific proteins, such as prostate-specific antigen (PSA), prostatic acid phosphatase, prostate-specific membrane antigen, probasin, and other human glandular kallikreins to drive the expression of therapeutic genes, treatment potentially can be targeted to prostate cancer cells throughout the body using a systemic approach.

Numerous potentially therapeutic genes and delivery systems are currently being developed and evaluated. Overall, the different gene therapy modalities can be grouped into three main categories: immunomodulators, corrective, and cytoreductive. Immunomodulation, just stated, attempts to augment the body's immune response to improve the immune system's natural ability to seek out and destroy cancer cells.

Corrective gene therapy which is already being used by many investigators in the treatment of patients with prostate cancer, involves the replacement or inactivation of a defective gene, such as a mutated tumor suppressor gene, or a dominant oncogene that has been found to play a role in the pathogenesis or progression of prostate cancer.

In November 2013, the results of a trial into a prostate cancer test called Polaris were announced in the UK.

It was happened at the National Cancer Research Institute conference. Cancer Research UK and other organizations supported the trial. It found that the test could measure the activity of particular genes (called cell cycle genes) in the prostate cancer cells. It can help doctors and researchers to know whether the cancer is a slow growing cancer that could safely be monitored. In addition, it could show whether the cancer is more quickly growing and so needs treatment.

Looking at the activity of the genes gives an overall cell cycle progression score (CCP score).It seems to be able to predict accurately whether the cancer will develop quickly or more slowly. However, doctors say that they still need to work out the best way of using this test to help patients. They need to find out how often to do a test to detect changes in gene activity. In addition, they need to shorten the time it takes to get the results. Therefore, this test is not currently available as a standard test for prostate cancer.

Tasquinimod clinical trials: This study was performed in collaboration with EXIN Diagnostics AB (public). Using automated software for analysis of the bone scan index (BSI) a quantitative measure of tumor burden in bone, the relation of the BSI with other prognostic biomarkers and overall survival were analyzed in a data set from the previously concluded Phase II tasquinimod clinical study. A delay in objective radiographic bone scan progression with tasquinimod using the BSI analysis was observed, and this delay is thought to be associated with improvements in survival.

Overall survival data from the randomized, placebo-controlled, double-blind clinical Phase II trial in approximately 200 men with metastatic castrate-resistant prostate cancer (mCRPC) was presented at 2012 ASCO Annual Meeting.

The intention to treat analysis showed median overall survival times (OS) of 33.4 vs. 30.4 months (p= 0.49, HR 0.87, 95% CI 0.59-1.29, ITT) in favor of tasquinimod, longer than previously reported in this metastatic prostate cancer population. A stronger trend for survival benefit is observed in patients with bone metastases; median OS was 34.2 vs. 27.1 months (p=0.19, HR 0.73, 95% CI 0.46-1.17). This phase II clinical trial was designed to test the safety and efficacy of tasquinimod. Noteworthy, 41 (61%) patients crossed-over from placebo to tasquinimod (mean time to crossover approximately. five months). In addition, there were imbalances in baseline prognostic factor in favor of the placebo arm.

These were addressed with a multivariate analysis of known CRPC prognostic factors.

It demonstrated a statistically significant OS advantage for tasquinimod treated patients with a hazard ratio (HR) of 0.64 (95% CI 0.42-0.97, p=0.034), a decrease of approximately 40% in the instantaneous risk of event (death) accompanied by improvement in progression-free survival (HR 0.52, 95% CI 0.35-0.78, p=0.001).

The primary endpoint in the Phase II trial was to show a difference in the number of patients with disease progression at six months. The results were published in the Journal of Clinical Oncology in October 2011 (please see publication list for full reference). Results showed that the fraction of patients who were disease progression-free after six months was 69% for patients treated with tasquinimod compared with 37% for placebo-treated patients (p<0.001). The median progression-free survival was 7.6 months for the tasquinimod group compared to 3.3 months for the placebo group (p=0.0042). Tasquinimod thus delayed disease progression by a median of 4.3 months. Tasquinimod treatment also had an effect on biomarkers relevant for prostate cancer progression and was well tolerated.

A pivotal Phase III trial 10TASQ10 is currently ongoing. The study is a global, randomized, double-blind, placebo-controlled trial in 1,245 patients with asymptomatic to symptomatic mCRPC. Criteria for study participation include diagnosed CRPC, presence of bone metastasis, evidence of progression after hormonal treatment, and no prior cytotoxic therapy for prostate cancer within two years. If the significant delay of disease progression reported in Phase II is confirmed in this Phase III trial, tasquinimod could further defer the use of more toxic chemotherapeutic treatments.

A Phase II proof-of-concept clinical trial is ongoing with the aim at establishing the clinical efficacy of tasquinimod used as maintenance therapy in patients with metastatic castrate-resistant prostate cancer (mCRPC) who have not progressed after a first-line docetaxel-based chemotherapy. Active Biotech's partner Ipsen also performs a new Phase II, proof-of-concept clinical trial with tasquinimod in a so-called umbrella study evaluating the compound in four different tumor types. The study evaluates the safety and efficacy of tasquinimod in advanced or metastatic hepatocellular, ovarian, renal cell and gastric carcinomas in patients who have progressed after standard therapies.

Tasquinimod mode of action: In order to grow and metastasize, tumors are dependent on successful interaction with the microenvironment at sites of growth. It includes formation and maintenance of a metastatic niche for tumor localization, blood vessels for nutrient and oxygen supply, as well as suppression of the local immune defense.

Preclinical studies have shown that tasquinimod's anti-prostate cancer efficacy involves its ability to interfere with all of these requirements. Tasquinimod has been shown to bind to the protein S100A9 that is present in tumor cells as well as different immune cells. This binding is believed to effect the composition of populations of different immune cells, which in turn will decrease immune suppression and angiogenesis.

Preclinical studies have concluded that tasquinimod exhibits anti-tumor activity via inhibition of tumor metastasis, angiogenesis, as well as modulation of immune cell populations.

Detection of Cancer Cells Directly

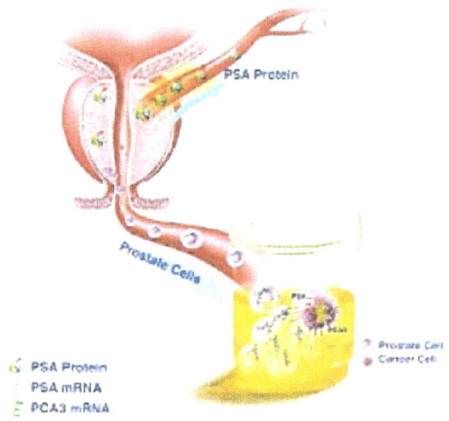

Diagram showing urinary PCA3 (lower arrow) vs serum PSA (upper arrow).Whereas PSA is a glycoprotein that may enter the bloodstream, PCA3 is a gene that exists in the nuclear material of prostate epithelial cells which may be shed into the urine. Those cells, if cancerous, over-express the gene. That over-expression, which may be many times that found in benign prostate cells, is detected by the assay. Importantly, PCA3 expression is normalized against a background of prostate specific nuclear material (PSAmRNA), yielding a PCA3 score.The PCA3 score is much more cancer-specific than serum PSA levels,which are confounded by factors such as prostate volume, age, trauma, and certain drugs.

CHAPTER 4

Tay-Sachs

In 1881 Warren Tay, a British ophthalmologist, found a "cherry red spot" in the retina of a one-year-old child with mental and physical retardation. Later, in 1896 Bernard Sachs, an American neurologist, noted extreme swelling of neurons in autopsy tissue from affected children. He also noted that the disease seemed to run in families of Jewish origin.

Both physicians were describing the same disease but it was not until the 1930s that the material causing the cherry-red spot and neuronal swelling was identified as a ganglioside lipid and the disease could be recognized as an "inborn error of metabolism." The term "ganglioside" was coined because of the high abundance of the brain lipid in normal ganglion cells (a type of brain cell). In the 1960s, the structure of the Tay-Sachs ganglioside was identified and given the name "GM2 ganglioside" (Figure 1).

Gangliosides are glycolipids. The lipid component, called ceramide, sits in the membranes of cells. Attached to it and sticking out into the extra-cellular space is a linked series of different sugars, the "glycol" portion of glycolipid. The essential function of gangliosides is not well understood, but they appear to have roles in biological processes as diverse as cell-to-cell recognition, differentiation, and in the repair of damaged neurons.

Gangliosides, like most cell components, are broken down and regenerated as part of normal cellular metabolism. The breakdown or "catabolism" of gangliosides occurs in the lysosome, a specialized vehicle that is analogous to the vacuole of plants. In the lysosome a series of acid hydrolases (degradative enzymes) removes each sugar, one at a time, until the ceramide lipid is all that remains. In Tay-Sachs disease, one of the lysosomal hydrolases, Hex A, is defective or completely absent, so the degradative process was blocked before completion. The result is the accumulation of G_{M2} ganglioside, the last molecule before the Hex A block in the catabolic sequence.

Since breakdown was blocked while synthesis continues, the result is a progressive accumulation of GM2 ganglioside and massive swelling of the lysosomes and hence of the neurons containing them. It is the basis of the neuron swelling observed by Sachs and the cherry-red spot described by Tay.

The cherry-red spot is due to the white appearance of swollen neurons of the retina surrounding the typically red fovea centralis (central depression in retina and site of maximum vision acuity) in the back of the eye (Figure 2).

Newborns with Tay-Sachs disease appear normal at birth. By six months of age, parents begin to notice that their infant is becoming less alert and is less responsive to stimuli. The affected infant soon begins to regress and shows increasing weakness, poor head control, and inability to crawl or sit. The disease continues to progress rapidly through the first years of life, with seizures and increasing paralysis. The child eventually progresses to a completely unresponsive vegetative state. Pneumonia often causes Death because of the child's weakened state. Some forms of Tay-Sachs disease are much milder with onset of the disease later in childhood or even adulthood. We now know that these forms of the disease are caused by less severe mutations in the *HEXA* gene.

 Introduced genetic engineering technique in the prevention of genetic diseases to the beginning of the 1990s...

 In 1989 an American woman gave birth to a child suffers from a rare disease and very strange known as (Tay-Sachs) affects members of the body and the brain as a result of a congenital defect inherited leads to the symptoms of severe and devastating ended in the death of the child and through examination of the father and mother found they sphere for gene causes the disease and thus the likelihood of injury to children arriving the same disease list resorted to a doctor in 1993 to test for genes can be made of the sperm that have been vaccinated ectopic father and mother through this test and sperm in the first test phase consisting of eight cells can be examined through gene know whether the child next suffering from the disease are disposed of sperm prior to their encampment, in the womb or sound completely fed sperm in the uterus for pregnancy and supplements the child is born naturally.. and the parents have agreed to conduct the experiment and examine the genes in the sperm cells of the eight have already been fertilized in vitro were taken from mother by spermatozoa father outside the uterus as is done in the case of a child pipes and when sperm were divided into eight cells were genetic testing shows that three of the embryos are completely free of disease genes (Tay) has been planting them and it was placed into the womb to grow and bigger, and nine months later was the birth of a healthy child for start a new page in the history of medicine is a change in the format and method of treatment for inherited diseases.

Tay-Sachs disease is a severe genetic disease of the nervous system that is nearly always fatal, usually by three to four years of age. It is caused by mutations in the *HEXA* gene, which codes for a component of the enzyme β-hexosaminidase A or "Hex A." The resulting accumulation of a brain lipid called G_{M2} ganglioside produces brain and spinal cord degeneration. It is a rare disease that is found in all populations, but it is particularly prevalent in Ashkenazi Jews of Eastern European origin. There is no treatment, but research aimed at treating the disease by blocking synthesis of the affected molecules has been ongoing since the late 1990s. Carriers can be identified by DNA or enzyme tests, and prenatal diagnosis is available to at-risk families.

A three years roadmap to gene therapy clinical trials for T-Sachs disease:

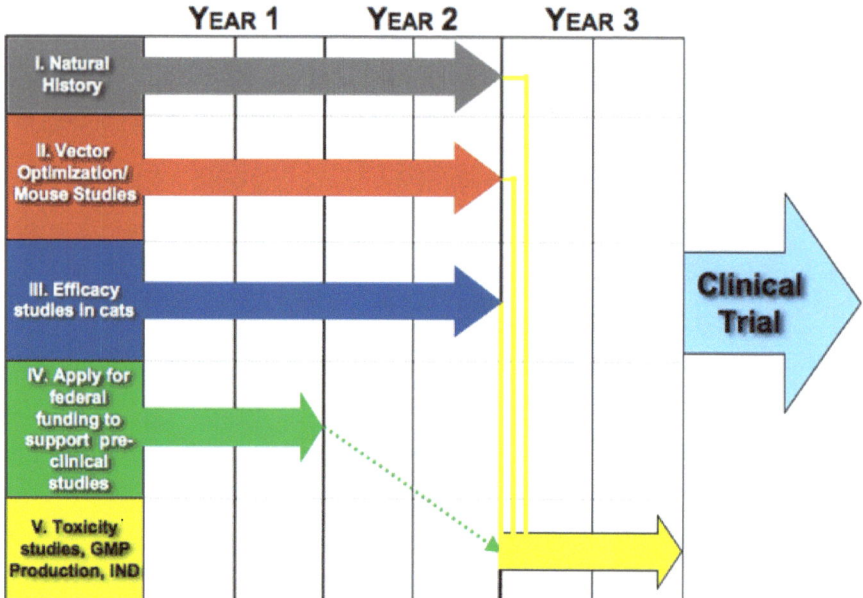

One in thirty Ashkenazi Jews is a carrier of one of the Tay-Sachs mutations. It is about ten times the frequency of carriers in non-Jews. Until 1970, it is estimated that about one in 4,000 births among Ashkenazi Jews was of a Tay-Sachs baby. It is producing a great desire to develop a carrier and prenatal test shortly after the enzyme defect was identified. Michael Kaback spearheaded a carrier-testing program that, by 2000, had tested well over 1 million Ashkenazi Jews, mainly in North America and Israel. It leads to a drop in the incidence of Tay-Sachs disease to less than one-tenth of its previous level.

The testing program has been so successful because it was organized through Jewish community groups, with the active participation of geneticists who conduct the tests. During the 1970s and 1980s, the test measured the level of Hex an activity in serum or white blood cells. With the identification of the Ashkenazi mutations, DNA testing came into use. Many geneticists prefer to conduct both types of tests, especially for non-Jews. They find DNA testing useful for its simplicity and exceedingly small error rate, but also recommend enzyme testing to guard against the involvement of a previously undetected mutation that would be missed by the mutation-specific DNA tests.

Future Prospects:

In the 1990s laboratories in the United States, Canada, and France developed mouse models of Tay-Sachs disease, Sand Hoff disease and G_{M2} activator deficiency. These investigations led to a much better understanding of the brain pathology and progression of the diseases.

A significant outcome has been the use of the mouse models to experiment with approaches to treatment. A promising approach is based on partially blocking the synthesis of gangliosides with drugs so that accumulation of G_{M2} ganglioside becomes minimal. In addition to "substrate deprivation," as this blocking action is called, other laboratories are trying gene therapy and drug-based methods for bypassing the Tay-Sachs defect.

The combination of carrier testing and prenatal diagnosis to assure the birth of healthy babies, and the more recent prospects for treating affected patients are significant advances since the discovery of a cherry red spot described in the first infant known to have been born with Tay-Sachs disease.

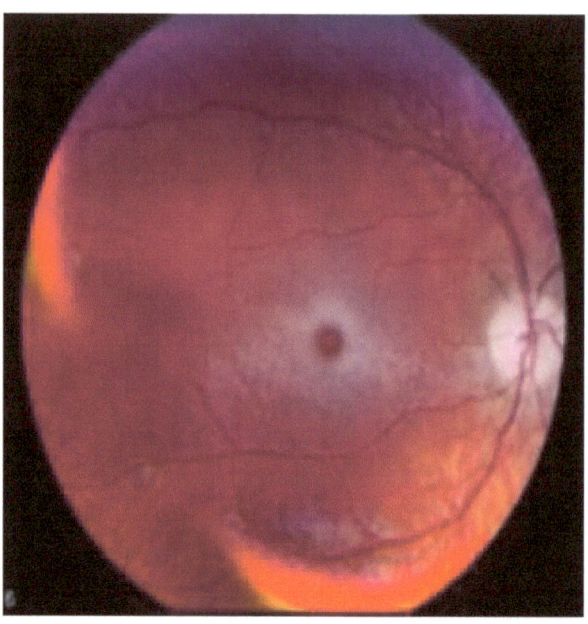

Tay-Sachs disease. Wikimedia Commons (Public Domain)

Brain with Tay-Sachs Disease

Hexosaminidase deficiency with accumulation of clear to foamy ganglioside neurons.

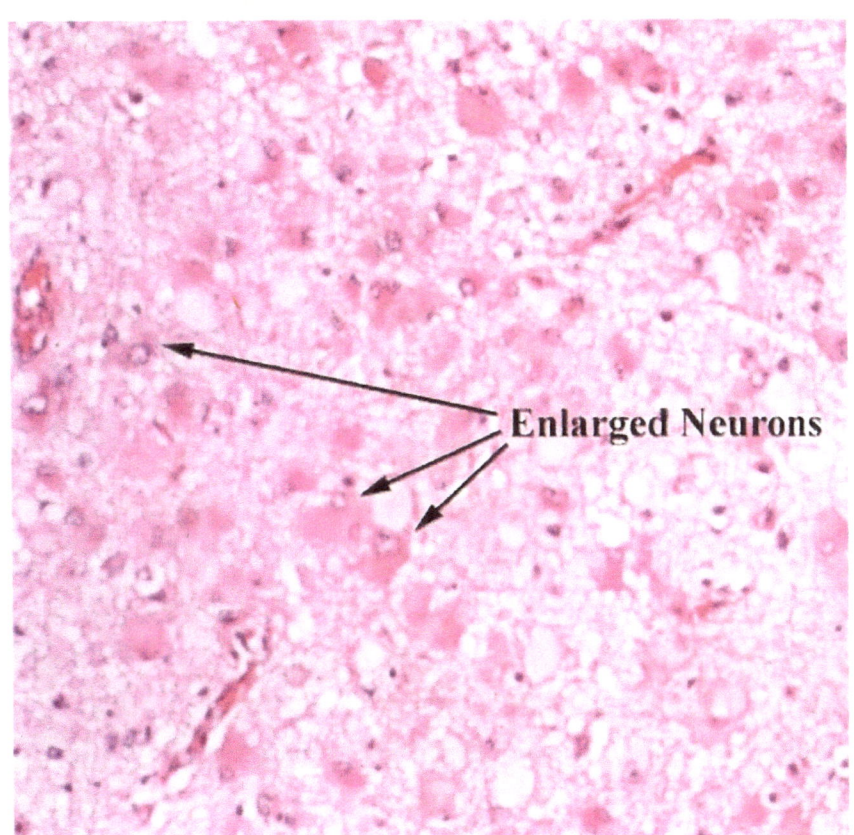

CHAPTER 5

Genetic Testing

More and more often, headlines boast of new cancer genes found.

No wonder people are left with many unanswered questions. What is the relationship between such gene discoveries and cancer? Is there a connection between genes and cancer's diagnosis or treatment? The answers to these and other gene questions lie in understanding gene discovery, the science behind gene testing the ability of researchers to identify changes within genes that may predict the future development of specific diseases, help diagnose existing diseases, or, someday, make it possible to treat or even ward off disease. Genetic tests have been designed for thousands of diseases. Most tests look at single genes and are used to diagnose rare genetic disorders, such as Fragile X Syndrome and Duchene Muscular Dystrophy. In addition, some genetic tests look at rare inherited mutations of otherwise protective genes, such as *BRCA1* and *BRCA2*, which are responsible for some hereditary breast and ovarian cancers. However, a growing number of tests are being developed to look at multiple genes that may increase or decrease a person's risk of common diseases, such as cancer or diabetes. Such tests and other applications of genomic technologies have the potential to help prevent common disease and improve the health of individuals and populations. For example, predictive gene tests may be used to help determine the risk of developing common diseases, and pharmacogenetic tests may be used to help identify genetic variations that can influence a person's response to medicines. There is much we still need to learn about how effective these new tests are, and the best way to use them to improve health. Gene testing involves examining a person's DNA--typically taken from cells in a sample of blood--for mutations linked to a disease or disorder.

Some genetic tests can identify changes in whole chromosomes. Others examine short stretches of DNA within genes. Others look for the protein products of genes.

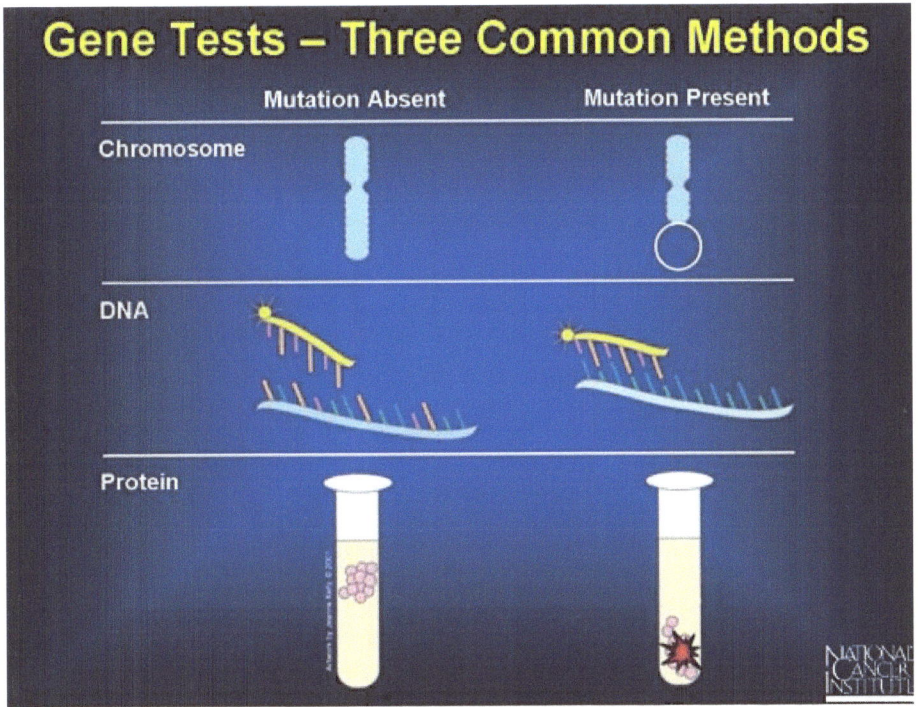

Despite the many scientific advances in genetics, researchers have only identified a small fraction of the genetic component of most diseases. Therefore, genetic tests for many diseases are developed based on limited scientific information and may not yet provide valid or useful results to individuals who are tested. However, many genetic tests are being marketed prematurely to the public through the Internet, TV, and other media. It may lead to the misuse of these tests and the potential for physical or psychological harms to the public.

 At the same time valid and useful tests, such as those for hereditary breast and ovarian cancer or for Lynch syndrome, a form of hereditary colorectal cancer, are not widely used, in part because of limited research on how to get useful tests implemented into practice across U.S. communities.

Genetic tests serve many purposes. They are widely used to screen newborns for a variety of disorders. Often this information enables the doctors to minimize the damage caused by the mutation.

In oncology, doctors use gene testing to diagnose cancer, to classify cancer into subtypes, or to predict a patient's responsiveness to new treatments.

Microarray Analysis: much of the excitement today centers on gene expression profiling that use a technology called microarrays. A DNA microarray is a thin-sized chip that has been spotted at fixed locations with thousands of single-stranded DNA fragments corresponding to various genes of interest. A single microarray may contain 10,000 or more spots, each containing pieces of DNA from a different gene. Fluorescent-labeled probe DNA fragments are added to ask if there are any places on the microarray, where the probe strands can match and bind. Complete patterns of gene activity can be captured with this technology.

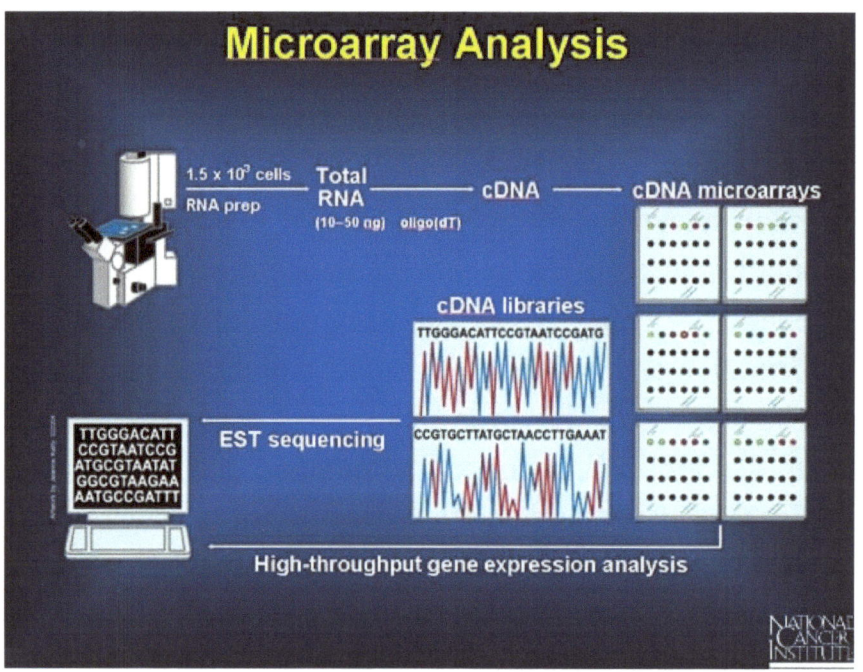

The scientists look for altered regions of the human genome--known DNA segments containing disease-linked mutations that are consistently inherited by persons with the disease and are *not found* in relatives who are disease free. Researchers use this information and tools from the Human Genome Project to zero in on the exact location of the altered gene or genes and characterize the specific base changes.

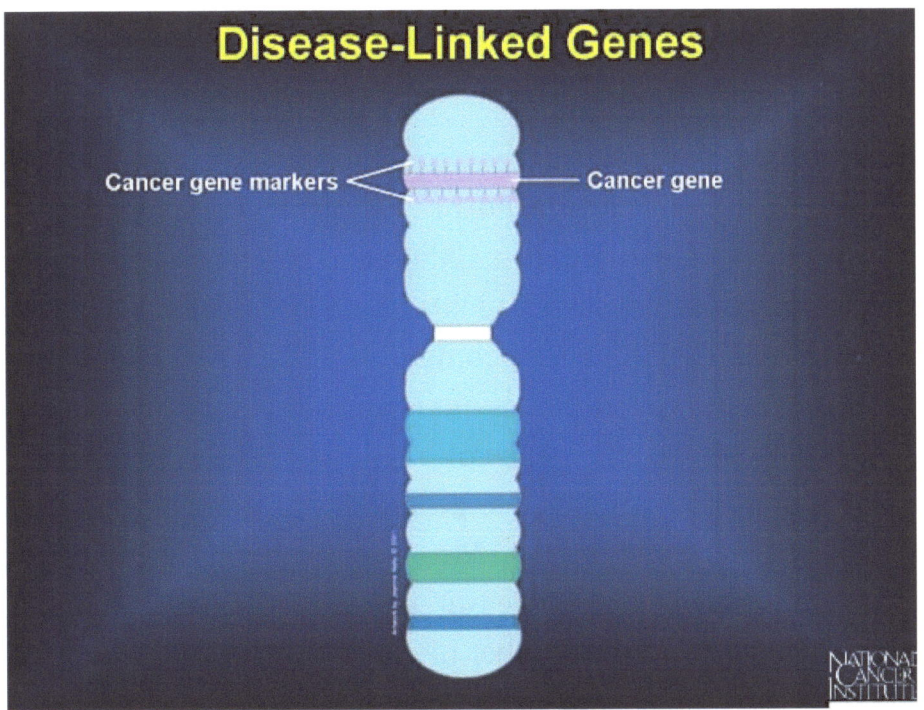

Disease-Linked Genes

Cancer gene markers

Cancer gene

Genetic Testing during Pregnancy: For genetic testing before birth, pregnant women may decide to undergo amniocentesis or chorionic villus sampling. There is also a blood test available to women to screen for some disorders. If this screening test finds a possible problem, amniocentesis or chorionic villus sampling may be recommended.

Amniocentesis is a test, usually, performed between weeks 15 and 20 of a woman's pregnancy. The doctor inserts a hollow needle into the woman's abdomen to remove a small amount of amniotic fluid from around the developing fetus. This fluid can be tested to check for genetic problems and to determine the sex of the child. When there is a risk of premature birth, amniocentesis may be done to see how far the baby's lungs have matured. Amniocentesis carries a slight risk of inducing a miscarriage.

Chorionic villus sampling (CVS) is, usually, performed between the 10th and 12th weeks of pregnancy. The doctor removes a small piece of the placenta to check for genetic problems in the fetus. Because chorionic villus sampling is an invasive test, there is a small risk that it can induce a miscarriage.

The genetic tests of the fastest growth areas in the science of medical diagnosis, thanks to the achievements of the draft HUMAN GENOM PROJECT have been identified, installation and isolate many of the genes responsible for hereditary diseases such as CYSTIC FIBROSIS anemia and HUNTINGTON CHOREA genetic commonly suffer from about 500 thousand people in the United States alone and who are asymptomatic at age forty or more through the emergence of bags and Vesicles in the kidneys, liver, pancreas and spleen and lead to inflation and possibly total renal failure involves genetic tests on a wide range of methods used to search for the existence of genes in cells or measurement .. and the effectiveness of these methods depends on the number of chromosomes in the cells of the patient or measuring the quantity of proteins in the blood of the patient Scouts or analyze genetic material of cells by molecular pathways can detect the genetic sequence qualitative one between three million pairs rules which form human genome material Currently there are four types of tests genetic:

1)AMINOCENTESIS : personal being tested after 10 weeks of pregnancy as taking some cells from the fluid tubercular order an examination to test the biological abnormality in the chromosomes . 2) CHORIONIC VILLUS SAMPLING: testing principles after ten weeks of pregnancy, where some cells take developing placenta countries to examine chromosomes. 3) COELOCENTESIS: talk test-not yet adopted-being before ten weeks of pregnancy.

Where some cells are taken from the cavity that surrounds the Earth and tubercular to examine chromosomes.

4) PREIMPLANTATION: test installation of genetic material (DNA) of the embryos at the stage of the eight cells to detect the presence of certain genetic defects. It allowed not genetic testing to preschool birth but can be used to diagnose genetic deformities in either children or adults. Applying these genetic tests can predict the course of the patient's health and warn of the danger of being sick...

In addition, if it was a combination of genetic tests hoped that the treatment the defective gene and gene functional sound, it would be able to these tests lead to a real cure.

Distinguishing features of the PCA3 assay (Gen-Probe, Inc.) are shown in sequence.

In **step No.1** (top), target capture of the mRNA is performed, using magnetic bead (purple).

In **step No. 2**, the captured gene is amplified using Transcription-Mediated Amplification, a process that generates some 10 billion copies of PCA3 in one hour.

In **step No. 3**, the Hybridization Protection Assay is performed using DNA probes tagged with a chemiluminescent substance that is activated upon contact with detection reagents. Details of the assay are described in a recent publication10.

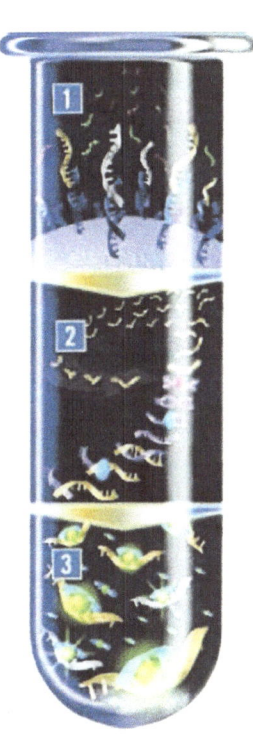

CHAPTER 6

Gene Treatment for Obesity

Obesity is a disorder characterized by an excess accumulation of body fat resulting from a mismatch between energy intake and expenditure. Incidence of obesity has increased dramatically in the past few years, almost certainly fuelled by a shift in dietary habits owing to the widespread availability of low-cost, hyper caloric foods. However, clear differences exist in obesity susceptibility among individuals exposed to the same obesogenic environment, implicating genetic risk factors. Numerous genes have been shown to be involved in the development of monofactorial forms of obesity. In genome-wide association studies, a large number of common variants have been associated with adiposity levels, each accounting for only a small proportion of the predicted heritability. Although the small effect sizes of obesity variants identified in genome-wide association studies currently preclude their utility in clinical settings, screening for a number of monogenic obesity variants is now possible.

Such regular screening will provide more prognoses that are informed and help in the identification of at-risk individuals who could benefit from early intervention, in evaluation of the outcomes of current obesity treatments, and in personalization of the clinical management of obesity.

This Review summarizes current advances in obesity genetics and discusses the future of research in this field and the potential relevance to personalized obesity therapy. The worldwide obesity epidemic has grave consequences because of increased risk of diabetes, cardiovascular disease, cancer, and other complications and reduced lifespan. Diet and exercise are the cornerstones of treatment, but an increasing number of patients will require therapeutic intervention to decrease and maintain body weight. Now a new *in vivo* work by Satya Kalra's group at the University of Florida shows that a gene therapy strategy has the potential to be tremendously useful as an obesity treatment in children.

To develop treatments for obesity, studies that help us understand the pathophysiology of body weight regulation are vital.

Such studies have shown that fat, rather than merely storing excess energy, also secretes substances that are actively involved in energy homeostasis as well as the complications of obesity.

Leptin is the best known of these substances. This hormone is secreted in proportion to body fat and regulates appetite and energy expenditure, mainly by influencing the brain.

Mutations of leptin or leptin receptor genes lead to overeating, impaired thermoregulation, massive weight gain, insulin resistance, diabetes, immune dysfunction, failure of sexual maturation and a variety of neuroendocrine abnormalities in rodents and humans. Conversely, recombinant leptin reverses these abnormalities in leptin-deficient animals. Leptin has also been implicated in the reproduction, angiogenesis, bone formation, brain development and regulation of the cardiovascular system. These diverse effects appear to occur mainly through the long leptin receptor and JAK-STAT signal transduction pathway.

The discovery of leptin created enormous excitement: surely, here was a simple way of treating obesity. However, it turned out that healthy animals are relatively insensitive to leptin. In fact, 'common' (diet-induced) obesity is typically associated with high circulating leptin and diminished sensitivity to peripheral leptin administration. Reduced transport of leptin to the brain and inhibition of leptin signal transduction are both possible causes of this reduction in sensitivity. Regardless, we still do not know if reduced leptin sensitivity is a cause or a consequence of obesity in most humans.

Gene therapy has been used to deliver leptin in genetically obese and normal rodents.Adeno-associated viruses (AAV) are ideal vehicles for leptin gene therapy as they are nonpathogenic, capable of infecting non dividing as well as dividing cells, and express the transgene over long periods. Using this technology, Karla and co-workers have previously demonstrated a prolonged reduction in body weight after injection of recombinant AAV virus encoding leptin (rAAV-leptin) in the brain (central leptin gene therapy). Presumably, central leptin gene therapy circumvents leptin resistance through a paracrine or autocrine process.

In 2001, six genes were linked to monogenic human obesity and no common variants were reproducibly associated with polygenic obesity. By 2008, progress in the field led to the discovery of eight monogenic genes and four polygenic genes (*FTO, PCSK1, MC4R, and CTNNBL1*) from associated studies at the genome-wide level of significance.

The recent emergence of the genome- wide association studies (GWAS) has led to further breakthroughs in gene identification and now nine loci are recognized to be involved in Mendelian forms of obesity along with 58 loci contributing to polygenic obesity.

In the new study published in *Pediatric Research*, a single injection of rAAV-leptin into the cerebral ventricle of immature rats prevented weight gain during the 10-month duration of the experiment. The treatment reduced food consumption as well as serum leptin, insulin and fatty acids, but increased uncoupling protein (UCP)-1 in brown adipose tissue (BAT) and ghrelin. The changes in BAT UCP-1 and ghrelin were observed in younger but not older animals. The authors analyzed mRNA levels of neuropeptides in the hypothalamus to understand the central actions of rAAV-leptin. NPY was decreased while proopiomelanocortin (precursor of α-MSH) was increased, suggesting that the reduction in appetite and body weight was mediated at least in part through hypothalamic neuropeptides. AGRP, a well-known leptin target that is localized in the arcuate nucleus with NPY, was not affected by central rAAV-leptin. Moreover, leptin gene therapy did not alter the timing of sexual maturation (vaginal opening) and duration of estrus cycles.

These new data clearly show that single injection of rAAV-leptin can achieve sustained weight reduction. Moreover, they demonstrate that this strategy can be used on immature animals without harming sexual maturation or reproductive cyclicity.

However, the mechanisms responsible for age-related differences in the response to rAAV-leptin, also found in other studies, need to be investigated. For example: why does rAAV-leptin have only a prolonged effect on food intake in younger animals, but not older animals? It seems that much of a long-term reduction in body weight is because of increased metabolic rate although the effect of leptin is diminished in older animals. In the latter case, activation of STAT-3 is healthy despite the reduced physiologic response to central rAAV-leptin, suggesting that age-related leptin resistance occurs through a mechanism downstream of leptin receptors and JAK-STAT pathway.

For a number of reasons, it is unlikely that these encouraging results are immediately applicable to humans. First, intrathecal administration of rAAV-leptin is not a practical mode of treatment in large populations. Second, while it has been reported that leptin is synthesized *de novo* in the brain, the long-term consequences of central rAAV-leptin on brain structure and function are not known. Third, the irreversibility of the rAAV-leptin and other gene therapy approaches raises safety and toxicity concerns. There are no in-built controls for expression of the rAAV-leptin transgene, so in some circumstances (e.g. after continuous leptin infusion) exposure to high leptin level can cause excessive weight loss with dire consequences in the long term. Theoretically, this obstacle may be overcome by placing the leptin gene under the control of a promoter responsive to signals involved in leptin regulation.

Traditional approaches for the management of overweight and obesity have proven poor long-term efficacy and obesity surgery is an efficient but invasive procedure. Prevention may, therefore, be considered as a promising strategy to face the obesity epidemic. In that context, the use of genetic information in clinical practice to predict individuals at high risk early in life and before the development of the disease remains the 'Holy Grail' for many geneticists. Is the current knowledge about obesity genetics, sufficient to envisage such translational medicine applications?

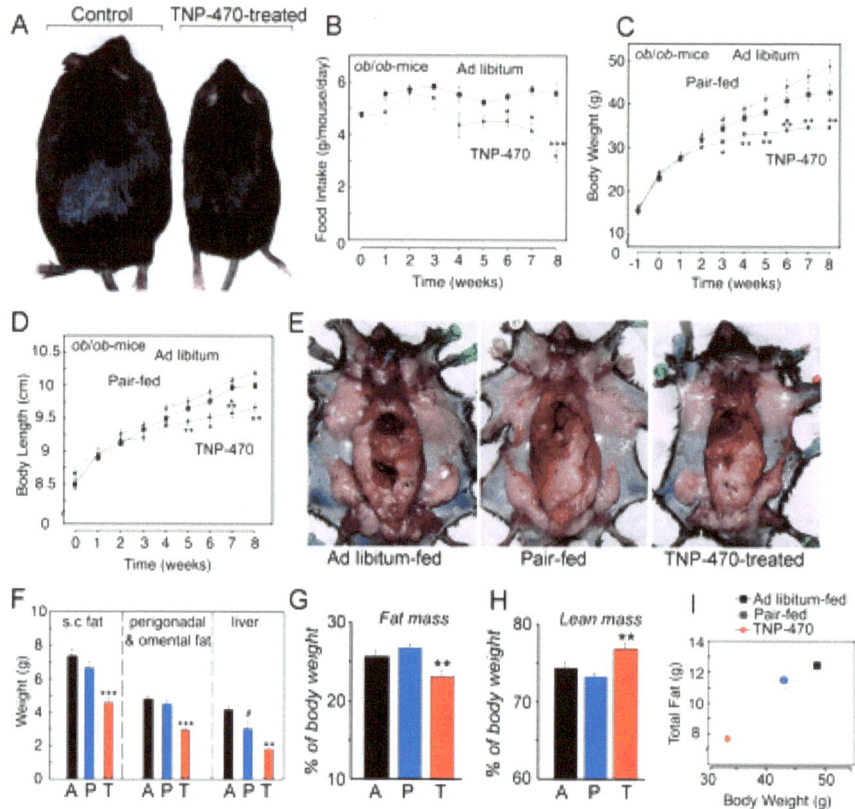

Figure 1. Prevention of obesity in *ob. /ob.* Mice by TNP-470. Five-week-old male C57Bl/6 *ob. /ob.* Mice were treated with TNP-470 at a dose of 20 mg/kg or received no treatment (A). Five-week-old male C57Bl/6 *ob. /ob.* Mice were treated with TNP-470 at a dose of 15 mg/kg. Ad libitum-fed and pair-fed mice were used as controls. Food intake was measured daily (B). Body weight was measured every other day (C) and body length once per week (D). Autopsy examination of adipose tissue distribution was performed at week 8 (E). Subcutaneous, perinatal, and omental fat depots and liver weights were measured (F). Total fat/total body weight (G), lean mass/total body weight (H), and the correlation between total fat mass versus body weight (I) was calculated. Black bars=ad libitum-fed mice (*A*), blue bars=pair-fed mice (*P*), red bars=TNP-470-treated animals (*T*). For comparisons with pair-fed group: *$P<0.05$, $P<0.01$, $P<0.001$; comparisons with ad libitum-fed group: #$P<0.05$.

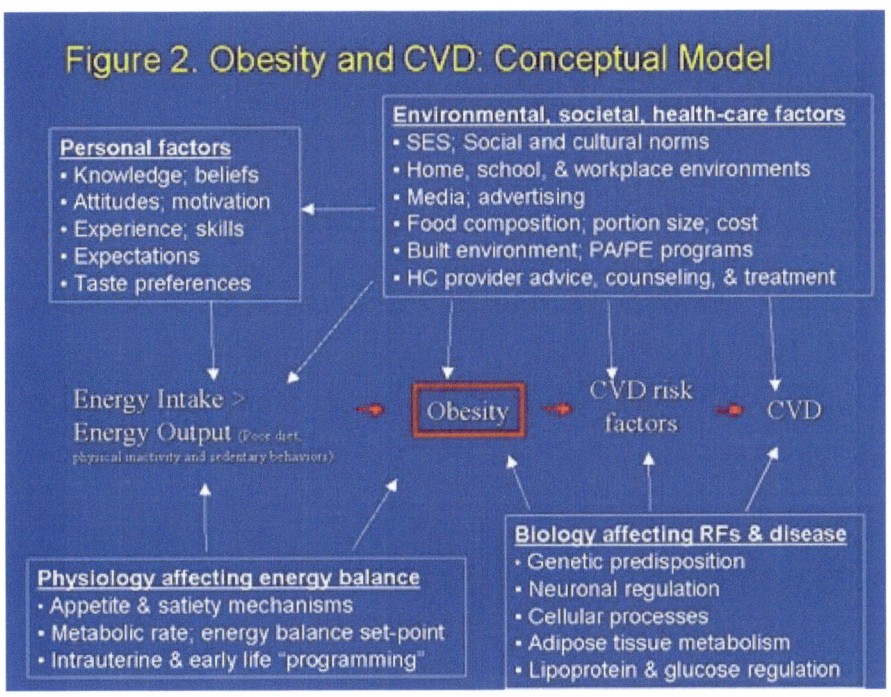

Figure 2. Obesity and CVD: Conceptual Model

Among the targets for the future treatment of genetic diseases following: 1) Hemophilia: People with hemophilia have low levels of certain blood clotting proteins, usually factor 8 or factor 9 (factor VIII or factor IX), which are necessary for clotting of the blood. These blood-clotting proteins are produced continually in a person without hemophilia.

Most of these proteins are produced in our livers. However, other cells contribute to the production also. Hemophilia is on the top of the list of disorders that may be cured with gene therapy because of its simplicity. It is only one missing blood clotting protein caused by one genetic mutation.

Hemophilia gene therapy should work like this. Scientist removes cells from a person with hemophilia. Usually, liver cells, but other cells, muscle, fat, etc. have proven to be successful. The scientists then alter the cells genetically by inserting new genetic material into them that reprograms the cells.

This new genetic material instructs the cells to produce factor 8 or 9 (factor VIII or factor IX). The cells are then reinserted into the person with hemophilia and viola! The person with hemophilia no longer has hemophilia.

Sounds simple, and there have been many successes with both animals & humans. There is an entire colony of dogs with hemophilia in Chapel Hill, North Carolina. There have also been many experiments with mice. There have also been several experiments with humans.

Hemophilia gene therapy works. The genetically altered cells produce factor. The cells survive and reproduce. Some of the 1990's experiments maintained factor levels for several months. Now the results are even more promising.

Some of the trials have maintained blood clotting factor levels for over three years and these trials are ongoing. These animals are still being studied. It is only a matter of time before these processes are perfected. The day will come when a person with hemophilia will go to a treatment center and leave without hemophilia.

Clotting factor concentrates can be made from human blood. The blood is treated to prevent the spread of diseases, such as hepatitis. With the current methods of screening and treating donated blood, the risk of getting an infectious disease from human clotting factors is very small; to further reduce the risk you or your child can take clotting factor concentrates that are not made from human blood. These are called recombinant clotting factors. Clotting factors are easy to store, mix, and use at home—it only takes about 15 minutes to receive the factor.

You may have replacement therapy on a regular basis to prevent bleeding. It is called preventive or prophylactic (PRO-fih-lac-tik) therapy.

Alternatively, you may only need replacement therapy to stop bleeding when it occurs. This use of the treatment, on an as-needed basis, is called demand therapy.

Need therapy is less intensive and expensive than preventive treatment. However, there is a risk that bleeding will cause damage before you receive the demand therapy.

Complications of replacement therapy include:

- Developing antibodies (proteins) that attack the clotting factor

- Developing viral infections from human clotting factors

- Damage to joints, muscles, or other parts of the body resulting from delays in treatment.

Researchers are trying to find ways to correct the faulty genes that cause hemophilia. Gene therapy has not yet developed to the point that it is an accepted treatment for hemophilia. However, researchers continue to test gene therapy in clinical trials.

Researchers at the UNC School of Medicine and the Medical College of Wisconsin found that a new kind of gene therapy led to a dramatic decline in bleeding events in dogs with naturally occurring hemophilia (A), a serious and costly bleeding condition that affects about 50,000 people in the United States and millions more around the world.

Before the gene treatment, the animals experienced about five serious bleeding events a year. After receiving the novel gene therapy, though, they experienced substantially fewer bleeding events over three years, as reported in the journal *Nature Communications*.

"The promise and the hope for gene therapy is that people with hemophilia would be given a single therapeutic injection and then would express the protein they are missing for an extended period of time, ideally for years or even their entire lifetimes," said Tim Nichols, director of the Francis Owen Blood Research Laboratory at UNC and co-author of the paper. The hope is that after successful gene therapy, people with hemophilia would experience far fewer bleeding events because their blood would clot better.

People with hemophilia a lack the coagulation factor VIII in their blood plasma -- the liquid in which red, white, and platelet cells are suspended.

"Bleeding events in hemophilia are severe, and without prompt factor VIII replacement, the disease can be crippling or fatal," said Nichols, a professor of medicine and pathology. "The random and spontaneous nature of the bleeding is a major challenge for people with hemophilia and their families."

In underdeveloped countries, people with hemophilia and many undiagnosed people typically die from bleeding in their late teens or early 20s. In developed countries, patients, usually, live normal lives, as long as they receive preventive injections of recombinant protein therapy a few times a week. The disease requires life-long management that is not without health risks. The annual cost of medications alone is about $200,000 a year.

Nichols and David Wilcox from the Medical College of Wisconsin figured out a potential way around the antibody response in dogs with naturally occurring hemophilia A.

Using a plasmapheresis machine and a blood-enrichment technique, the research team isolated specific platelet precursor cells from three dogs that have hemophilia A. The team then engineered those platelet precursor cells to incorporate a gene therapy vector that expresses factor VIII.

The researchers put those engineered platelet precursors back into the dogs. As the cells proliferated and produced new platelets, more and more were found to express factor VIII.

Then, nature took over. Platelets naturally discharge their contents at sites of vascular injury and bleeding. In this experiment, the contents included factor VIII.

Several new technologies are also being implemented to advance hemophilia treatment. These new technologies, once used to destroy viruses in blood, have been successful in virtually eliminating the risk of contracting HIV or hepatitis C from clotting factor today. Pharmaceutical companies are continuing to investigate genetically manufactured product alternatives derived from little to no human blood products. New products have consistently been developed that have an even higher purity than previously available.

It is important to mention that emerging therapeutic advances should not be justified or brought to market based only on the notion that they will be more affordable, although that might be the case, but also, and more importantly that they will be therapeutically more advantageous.

Improvements in treatment adherence, reductions in bleeding frequency (including micro hemorrhages), better management of trough levels, and improved health outcomes (including quality of life) should be the foremost considerations.

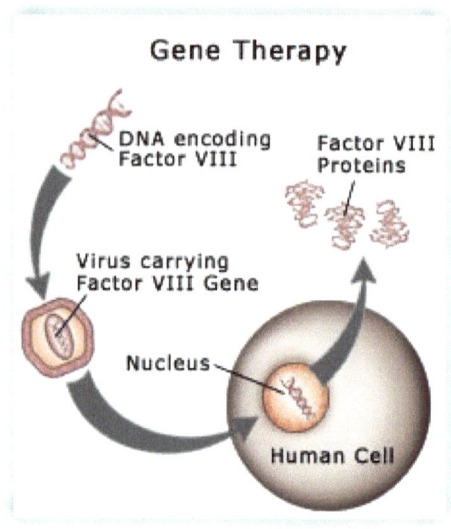

Gene therapy

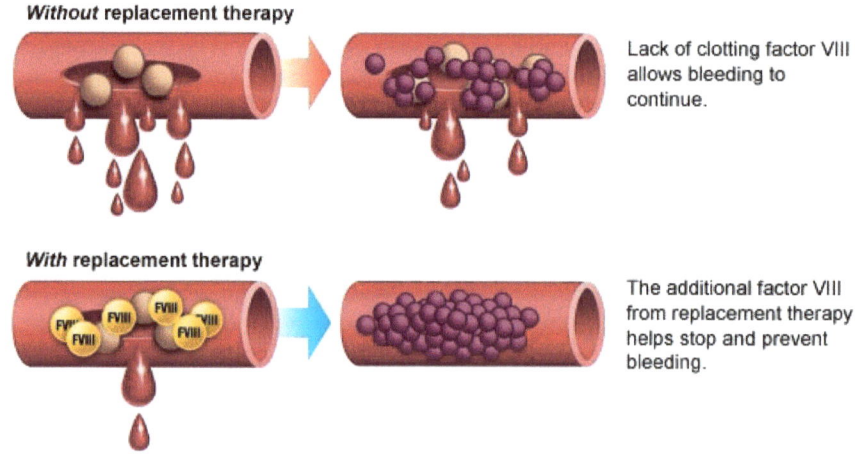

2) Diabetes: Diabetes mellitus is, usually, classified as type 1 or type 2 diabetes. Type 1 results from a β-cell defect, often due to an autoimmune process. Type 2 diabetes is characterized by insulin resistance, which is often combined with an insulin secretory defect. The number of people suffering from diabetes is growing at an alarming rate. In 1997, the

estimated number of people worldwide with diabetes was 124 million, 97% of these having type 2 diabetes. Based on estimates of changes in lifestyle, economic development and population figures, the global prevalence of diabetes mellitus by the year 2010 is projected to reach 221 million people. Since severe complications can occur if the disease is not under strict glycemic control, it is evident that the epidemic of diabetes is becoming an enormous health problem.

In the light of this disturbing scenario not only are efforts to promote exercise and low-fat intake of paramount importance, but also new techniques that can restore metabolic control in a safe and cost-efficient manner must be developed. One such approach, which might be useful, is gene therapy.

The using a broad definition of gene therapy, it is possible to outline quite a few gene transfer strategies that could help diabetics.

The DNA sequence of the treatment works by sensing an increase in glucose concentrations in the body (such as after a meal) and then with the help of a glucose inducible response element (GIRE), prompts the injected DNA to produce insulin, similar to the way normal pancreatic cells do. Instead of targeting pancreatic cells, the therapy exclusively targets the liver (the liver as the ideal target for this therapy because of its ability to regenerate).

In order for the therapy to be effective, the DNA needs to enter and attach to millions of cells, so the liver's ability to replace dead cells was an obvious advantage. The treatment essentially makes the liver function like a mini-pancreas."

Type 1 diabetes mellitus results from the autoimmune destruction of insulin-producing cells of the pancreas. There is no cure for T1DM; insulin therapy, which must be given multiple times per day, is the sole active treatment. Although injectable insulin preserves life, maintaining glucose control is difficult to do and often causes chronic hyperglycemia, which can lead to end-stage kidney failure, blindness, and amputations.

Based on serum lipid profiles and other markers of liver function, the study showed that a single treatment adequately protected the diabetic rats from many of the long-term diabetes-associated damage.

Gene and cell therapy scientists are developing methods to reprogram some of the other cells of the pancreas to secrete insulin. Currently, ongoing clinical trials using these gene and cell therapy strategies hold promise for improved treatments of type I diabetes in the future.

Gene therapy scientists are investigating the optimal and safest method for transferring an efficiently expressing insulin gene into other cells, including those in the liver, stomach, or intestines. Induced pluripotent stem cells (iPSCs) have been isolated from type 1 diabetic subjects; they are a useful tool to study disease mechanism. Furthermore, different laboratories are trying to develop efficient protocols to induce the differentiation of iPSCs into beta-like cells. These studies are currently being conducted in vitro and animals and not yet in clinical trials.

The main challenges for this approach include, (1) achieving the proper regulation of expression by the insulin gene to make the proper amount of insulin, and (2) avoiding a repeated aberrant immune response to these gene-modified cells, an autoimmunity that previously resulted in the killing of the patient's insulin-producing beta cells.

Alternatively, other preclinical studies are investigating gene-based therapies to overcome the patient's aberrant immune response to pancreatic beta cells through the delivery of genes encoding immune suppressive proteins, called cytokines, such as TGF-beta and interleukin 10 into the pancreas, which in turn may suppress this autoimmune response allowing the patient's own insulin-secreting beta cells to survive.

Furthermore, the pancreas also contains other cells called exocrine cells, which secrete digestive enzymes. Significantly, these cells remain intact in patients with type 1 diabetes and thus, could potentially be gene modified to secrete insulin as an alternative genetic approach to treating this disease. Recently, gene therapy researchers have identified three genes that can convert adult pancreatic exocrine cells into pancreatic beta cells. In preclinical animal models, these reprogrammed exocrine cells were identical to beta cells in size, shape and expression of essential genes, and resulted in reduced blood sugar levels and improved sugar distribution. Other cells that have been shown to be susceptible to reprogramming to become beta-like cells include pancreatic alpha cells, pancreatic ductal cells and adult stem cells in the liver.

In addition to gene transfer strategies, a variety of cell therapy approaches is also being investigated for the treatment of type 1 diabetes. Multiple clinical trials are currently recruiting patients to assess the ability of transplantation of various cell populations to normalize blood sugar levels, reduce disease symptoms, and assess safety. Some tests utilize patient-derived cells (termed autologous cells) for therapy while others utilize donor-derived cells (termed allogeneic cells) obtained from other humans.

Currently, there are over 20 ongoing human clinical trials utilizing one of the following cell sources to transfer or generate pancreatic beta cells in patients with type I diabetes, allogeneic pancreatic beta cells, mesenchymal stem cells, cord blood stem cells, or autologous adipose-derived stem cells.

Several cell therapy trials also include different regimens of immunosuppressive medications designed to abrogate the aberrant anti-beta cell autoimmune response, and specific nutrients (vitamin D, omega 3 fatty acids which are usually low in diabetics) designed to improve clinical outcomes and reduce side effects. In addition, several clinical studies testing the ability of distinct cell populations to reduce the immune response against the beta cells are currently ongoing. Furthermore, ongoing studies using either autologous or allogeneic hematopoietic stem cell transplant, with an aim to delete beta cell targeted autoimmune cells may additionally provide promising data to expanding this approach further either alone or in combination with other gene and cell-based approaches to treat patients with type I diabetes. Collectively, these multiple genes and cell-based approaches represent the advent of a new and promising era in diabetes research.

As promising preclinical studies mature into clinical studies and as the multiple ongoing clinical studies accrue data, there are clear signs that these novel gene and cell based innovative approaches hold real promise for advanced and improved treatment strategies for patients with type I diabetes.

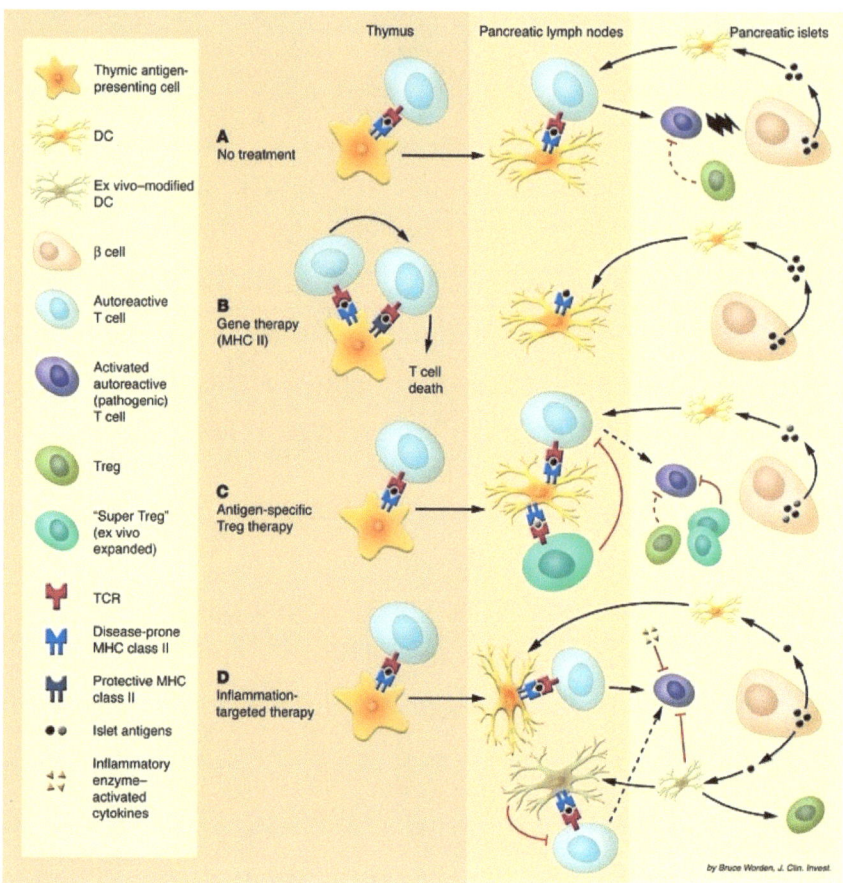

(A) Due to several combined defects, auto reactive T cells in NOD mice escape negative selection in the thymus and become activated in the pancreatic lymph nodes. The resulting effector T cells are kept under control for a limited period (resulting in peri-insulitis) until regulation (likely to involve Treg's) is no longer sufficient, and overt T1DM develops. (B) In irradiated NOD mice reconstituted with HSCs expressing a protective form of MHC class II, auto reactive T cells are efficiently deleted in the thymus, and no insulin is observed. (C) Antigen-specific Treg's from the islet infiltrate may be isolated and expanded ex vivo. When reintroduced, these cells prove to be efficient suppressors and may do so both in the pancreatic lymph nodes and the pancreatic lesions, (D) DCs or antigen-specific T cells) may be isolated and modified ex vivo to express: (a) immunoregulatory proteins that induce tolerance, apoptosis, or immune deviation of auto reactive T cells; and (b) appropriate receptors to enhance their trafficking into the sites of inflammation. Alternatively, inhibitory cytokines that have been engineered to become activated only under inflammatory conditions can be injected. These two strategies favor local versus systemic action of inhibitory products.

CHAPTER 7

Genetic Engineering and the Environment

"Environment" is defined as our surroundings that include the abiotic component (the non-living) and biotic component (the living) around us. The abiotic environment includes water, air and soil while the biotic environment consists of all living organisms – plants, animals and microorganisms. Environmental pollution broadly refers to the presence of undesirable substances in the environment that are harmful to man and other organisms. In the past decade or two, there has been a significant increase in the levels of environmental pollution mostly due to direct or indirect human activities. With the simultaneous increase in cases of cancer, autoimmune diseases, and infections caused by antibiotic-resistant microorganisms, the healthcare system was left depleted of professionals able to manage the situation. Biotechnology is being used to provide alternative cleaner technologies, which will help further to reduce the hazardous environmental implications of the traditional technologies. E.g., some Fermentation technologies have some serious environmental implications. Various biotechnological processes have been devised in which all nutrients introduced for fermentation are retained in the final product, which ensures high conversion efficiency and low environmental impact.

In a paper industry, the pulp bleaching techniques are being replaced by more environmentally-friendly technologies involving biotechnology. The pulp processing helps to remove the lignin without damaging valuable cellulosic fibers, but the available techniques suffer from the disadvantages of high costs, high-energy use and corrosion.

A lignin-degrading and modifying enzyme (LDM) was isolated from *Phanerochaete chrysosporum* and was used, which on one hand, helped to reduce the energy costs and corrosion and on the other hand increased the life of the system. This approach helped in reducing the environmental hazards associated with bleach plant effluents.

In Plastic industry, the conventional technologies use oil-based raw materials to extract ethylene and propylene, which are converted to alkene oxides and then polymerized to form plastics such as polypropylene and polyethylene.

There is always the risk of these raw materials escaping into the atmosphere thereby causing pollution. Using biotechnology, safer raw materials as if sugars (glucose) are being used which are enzymatically or through the direct use of microbes converted into alkene oxides.e.g. *Methylococcus encapsulates* has been used for converting alkene into alkene oxides.

INTEGRATION OF BIOLOGICAL STEPS IN PULPING PROCESS LEADING TO LIGNIN DEGRADATION

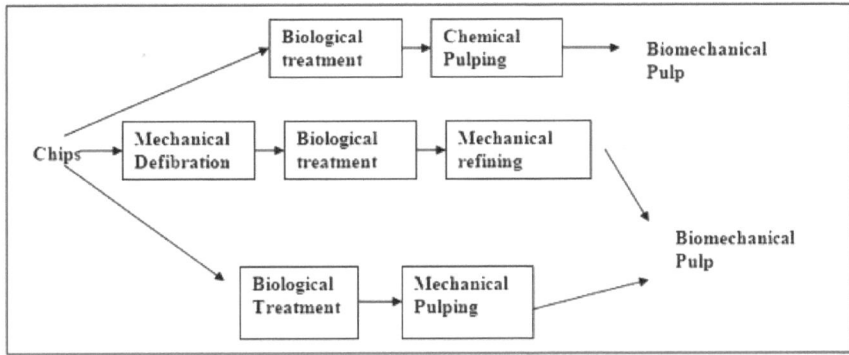

In the last century, thanks to the development of molecular trials such as those involving genetic modification, biotechnologies have asserted themselves in diversified sectors and their evolution has been rapid, resulting in an enormous impact on the productive sector, on the quality of life, and on the consequences that their employment can have for man and, above all, for the environment.

In particular, the application of biotechnologies in the area concerned with the management and disposal of dangerous and non-dangerous wastes as well as in the sector concerned with the remediation of grounds contaminated by organic and inorganic pollutants, has led to the development of systems and processes that represent a valid and consolidated methodology for environmental improvement.

Every day new developments emerge and impressive achievements in the field of technology, an area vital research... I mean trying to improve the capabilities of living organisms through pooling characteristics of many types are often very different. The game is moving genes from one organism to be separated and injected in the cell of another organism. To become cell more new capacity to produce different vehicles or to carry out controversial surprisingly has never exercised over the years. It is precisely the essence of genetic engineering and sinew...

A synthetic material for a plastic, for example, has become an important part in our lives is hard to ignore, since it was well... Recent research has paid attention to try to produce new vehicles similar in denaturalization vehicles Plastic. However, it difficult the microbial digestion... So that the closure of one life cycles. Indeed, the researchers find a chemical empire in England to discover one super strains layers ability to convert sugar to (polyester) in the semi-bacterial qualities natural plastic material mostly. The scientists used genetic engineering this miracle microbe and went on to develop through the transfer of new genetic mechanism to ensure production and abundant (polyester) promised to replace the plastic.

The really surprising that ecologists have expressed their welcome new microbe, it is a digestible bacterial mere samples of it buried in the soil, to break away completely after a period similar to the period required to analyze the paper.

We have sent a science of genetic engineering scientists hope to the environment in the production of alternative materials for synthetic materials, but materials are natural microbial digestion and entry into the natural life cycle without pollution.

Phytoextraction: the use of plant to take up metal contaminants from soil through the absorption by plant roots. The metal absorbed are stored or accumulated in the aerial portions of the plants (Stems & Leaves). Plants intended for this application are called hyper accumulators. These species of plants have a high tolerance to heavy metals and are capable of absorbing larger amount of metal in comparison to other plants. Today, researchers are developing genetically engineered hyper accumulators that have a higher metal accumulation and tolerance capacity.

After the plants are allowed to absorb the contaminants for some time, they are harvested to be either disposed of by incineration or be composted to recycle metals.

Although plants that were incinerated will be disposed off in a hazardous waste landfill, the amount of the plant ash generated will be below 10% of the volume that would be produced if contaminated soil were excavated for treatment.

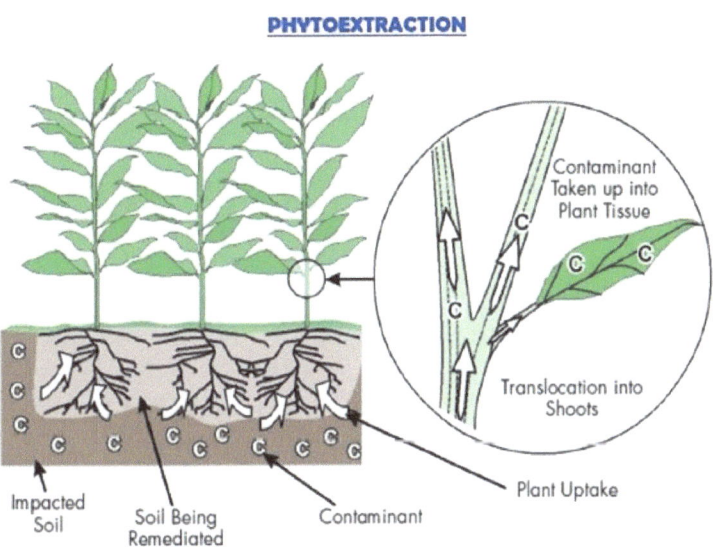

The plants take up the contaminant through the system of roots and store them in the roots or transport them up into the stems and leaves. The plants will carry on absorbing contaminants until it is being harvested. After the harvest, the soil will contain a lower concentration of a contaminant. As such, this growth and harvest cycle is, usually, repeated for a number of times to achieve a considerable clean up. After the process, the remediated soil can be put into other beneficial uses.

Gene to improve phytoextraction: problem in the use of phytoaccumulation is that they do not have enough biomass and growth rate to be applied in large-scale practices to resolve this problem, phytoextraction can be further improved by transfer of genetic traits from the hyper accumulator into plants that have high biomass and growth rate. In this way, plants with high biomass and growth rate will also take up large quantity of metals.

For example, Poplar and willow do not accumulate metals to the high concentration. However, they are still active mediators because of their deep root system and biomass. Hence, they became excellent candidate to be genetically engineered to have traits of hyper-accumulators.

Metals accumulated pose a significant risk to consumers of plants. As such, plants capable of producing substances that deter or discourage herbivores from feeding them can be transformed to have improved metal tolerance and capabilities. With such a system in place, it will help prevent the transfer of metals to the food chain.

Transfer of gene extracted from bacteria or animals into plants systems are attempts to improve the potential of remediation. Some bacteria have the genetic characteristic to detoxify toxic elements. Today, the transfer of such genes into plants had already produced promising results.

For instances, no plants have been shown to be able to tolerate some elements such as mercury or lead. It can be changed by transferring genes from bacteria that can detoxify these metals (mercury & lead) into plants. With the transfer of the expressing gene, plants can be genetically altered to be used clean up these metals, which were once seemed to be impossible.

The use of transgenic plants also addresses the problem of the mix contamination that is happening in a polluted site. Methods, which involve introducing several genes at once into plants, have help in the removal of complex and mixed pollutants.

CHAPTER 8

Genetic Engineering and Pollution Problem

Environmental pollutants such as heavy metals and pesticides are commonly present in water emanating from acid mine drainage or other industries and agricultural runoffs. These toxic pollutants can accumulate in living organisms and produce the adverse effects such as carcinogenicity and acute toxicity. Complete mineralization and removal of these pollutants and their toxic byproducts can be achieved using a biological process that uses active bacterial/fungal/mixed microbial cultures.

Bacteria have a well-earned reputation for causing disease, but now certain types of microorganisms are being put to good use by improving water cleanliness and safety.

Wastewater produced by factories is contaminated with heavy metals—elements that are naturally present in our bodies in small amounts, but which can be extremely dangerous to humans at higher levels of concentration.

For cleaning, this industrial wastewater, it will put through the process of bioremediation, or the use of microorganisms to treat water that has been contaminated by hazardous materials. Water that has been cleaned by this method can then be released into the environment or even reused.

One method of bioremediation is called biogenic hydrogen sulfide precipitation technology.

Research conducted by the National Institute of Molecular Biology and Biotechnology (BIOTECH) of the University of the Philippines at Los Baños found that this strategy can treat and remove heavy metal contaminants such as copper, lead, zinc and chromium from industrial waste water at the laboratory level.

These findings were relayed by BIOTECH researcher, Dr. Lorele Trinidad at a seminar organized by the DOST in conjunction with National Biotechnology Week in November 2011 at the Department of Environment and Natural Resources compound in Diliman, Quezon City.

The Philippine Council funded the institute's research for Industry Energy and Emerging Technology Research and Development of the Department of Science and Technology (DOST-PCIEERD). The towns of Marilao, Meycauayan and Obando in Bulacan participated in the project; effluents from local gold smelting and tanning industries had polluted their river system.

DOST Secretary Mario G. Montejo believes that biotechnological methods such as bioremediation can be powerful tools in addressing many of our issues, including ensuring water safety and protecting the health of Filipinos.

"Today's society faces lingering and emerging challenges, underscoring the importance of utilizing new and proven technologies in developing solutions.

Microbial consortia have been shown to be more suitable for bioremediation of recalcitrant compounds such as pesticide residues as their biodiversity supports environmental survival and increases the number of catabolic pathways available for contaminant biodegradation. In the case of heavy metal contaminated wastewaters, bio sorption has emerged as a promising low-cost methodology wherein biological catalysts are employed to remove and recover heavy metals from aqueous solutions.

The metal removal mechanism is a complex process that depends on the chemistry of metal ions, cell wall compositions of microorganisms, physiology of the organism, and physicochemical factors like pH, temperature, time, ionic strength, and metal concentration.

Treatment of sewage using microorganisms:

The sewage is defined as the wastewater resulting from the various human activities, agriculture and industries and mainly contains organic and inorganic compounds, toxic substances, heavy metals and pathogenic organisms. The sewage is treated to get rid of these undesirable substances by subjecting the organic matter to biodegradation by microorganisms. The biodegradation involves the degradation of organic matter to smaller molecules (CO_2, NH_3, PO_4 etc.) and requires a constant supply of oxygen. The process of supplying oxygen is expensive, tedious, and requires a lot of expertise and manpower. Growing microalgae in the ponds and tanks where sewage treatment is carried out overcome these problems. The algae release the O_2 while carrying out the photosynthesis, which ensures a continuous supply of oxygen for biodegradation.

The algae are also capable of adsorbing certain heavy toxic metals due to the negative charges on the algal cell surface, which can take up the positively charged metals. The algal treatment of sewage also supports fish growth, as algae are a good source of food for fishes. The algae used for sewage treatment are *Chlorella, Euglena, Chlamydomonas, Scenedesmus, Ulothrix, Thribonima, etc.*

As the majority of genes responsible for the synthesis of enzymes with biodegradation capacity are located on the plasmids, the genetic manipulations of plasmids can lead to the creation of new strains of bacteria with different degradative pathways. In 1970s, Chakrabarty and his team of co-workers reported the development of a new strain of bacterium Pseudomonas by manipulations of plasmid transfer, which they named as "superbug". This superbug had the capability of degrading a number of hydrocarbons of petroleum simultaneously such as camphor, octane, xylene, naphthalene, etc. In 1980, United States granted the patent to this superbug making it the first genetically engineered microorganism to be patented.

In certain cases, the process of plasmid transfer was used. E.g., the bacterium containing CAM (camphor degrading) plasmid was conjugated with another bacterium with OCT (octane degrading) plasmid. Due to non-compatibility, these plasmids cannot coexist in the same bacterium. However, due to the presence of homologous regions of DNA, recombination occurs between these two plasmids which results in a single CAM-OCT plasmid giving the bacterium the capacity to degrade both camphor, as well as octane.

A new strain of Pseudomonas sp. (strain ATCC 1915) has been developed for the degradation of the vanillate (which is a waste product from the paper industry) and sodium dodecyl sulfate (SDS, a compound used in detergents).

The Fraunhofer Institute for Interfacial Engineering and Biotechnology IGB and its European partners have developed several efficient methods for eliminating persistent pollutants from wastewater. Some of these processes generate reactive species, which can be used to purify even highly polluted landfill leachate while another can also remove selected pollutants, which are present in very small quantities with polymer-adsorbed particles.

Open plasma processes for water purification: Another new approach for purifying water involves the use of atmospheric pressure plasma. Plasma is an ionized gas containing not only ions and electrons but also chemical radicals and electronically excited particles as well as short wave radiation. Plasma can be ignited by means of an electromagnetic field e.g. by applying high voltage. The plasma glow is characteristic and can be seen in the fluorescent lamps of neon signs used for advertising purposes. In a technical sense, plasma processes have already been used specifically for modifying and cleaning surfaces for a long time now.

This principle is currently being applied by the partners of a joint water plasma project, funded by the EU, entitled "Water decontamination technology for the removal of recalcitrant xenobiotic compounds based on atmospheric plasma technology", grant agreement no. 262033, www.waterplasma.eu, in which a plasma is used for purifying water in an oxidative process. The result is a plasma reactor in which the reactive species formed in the plasma can be transferred directly to the contaminated water. The reactor is "open" so that the plasma is in direct contact with the flowing water film.

The plasma reactor is designed in such a way that plasma can be ignited and maintained between a grounded electrode in the form of a stainless steel cylinder within the reactor and a copper network acting as high voltage electrode.

To do that, high voltage is applied. The copper network is on a glass cylinder which acts as a dielectric barrier, also shielding the reactor to the outside. Polluted water is pumped upwards through the stainless steel cylinder in the center of the plasma reactor. When the water flows down the outer surface of the cylinder, it passes through the plasma zone between the stainless steel cylinder and the copper network where the pollutants are oxidized.

In laboratory experiments, Fraunhofer researchers were able to discolor a methylene blue solution completely within a few minutes. Cyanide was also broken down effectively by 90 percent within only 2 minutes. Based on such promising results, the process is now being tested on a larger scale. One of the project partners is working with a demonstrator, which can purify 240 liters of contaminated water in one hour. The results will be used to continually optimize the design of the reactor and its process controls. The ultimate aim is to bring the reactor to market together with further partners from industry. The open plasma process has a high potential because there is no barrier between the plasma, where the oxidative radicals are formed, and the contaminated water.

Systems solutions for water supply and water treatment: These innovative processes for water treatment complement the Fraunhofer IGB's portfolio in the fields of water purification and water treatment.

Together with further processes for water treatment and recovering wastewater components as energy and fertilizing salts, the Fraunhofer IGB is steadily optimizing wastewater treatment plants and improving DEUS 21, a system for the semi-decentralized purification of household wastewater.

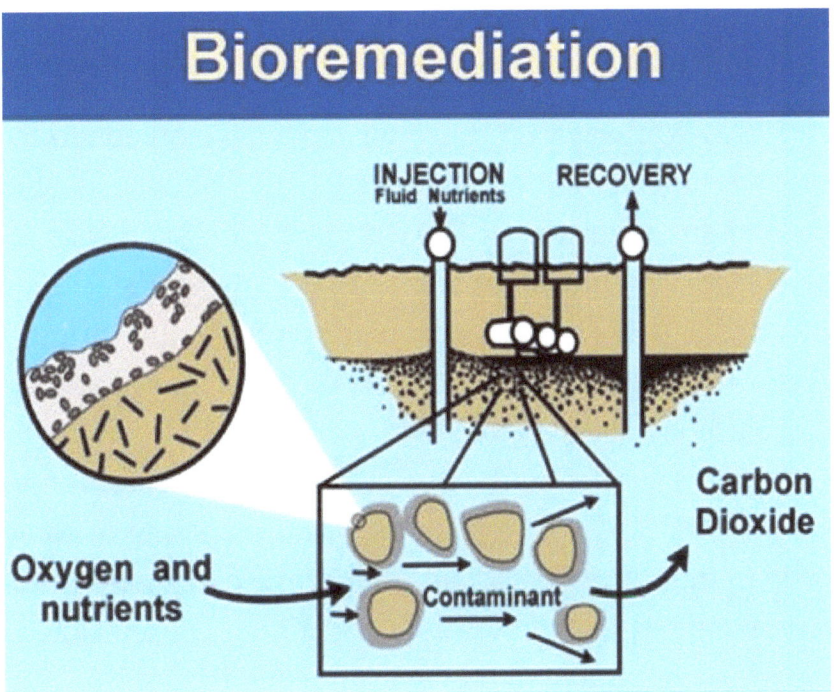

The global stock of freshwater cause for concern Thus, killing cries scientists demanding everyone's mind and conscience to preserve the precious drop of water.

But advocacy of the need to use water again and again through the life cycles of scientists has begun micro-organisms (microbiological) in Educational bacterial strains strange mood where not only grow in sewage , thus been reared in tanks inside those massive stores of water and then the bacteria feed on various solid waste and liquid However, these natural bacteria often those who rebel bad life in the sewage we see it strike on the analysis of all the waste and complete analysis then we can re-use water treatment only for the purpose of irrigation and agriculture.

Scientists, therefore, decided to genetic engineering to intervene with these organisms so willingly embrace of several genes and genetic new genotype within its video to make it more capable of swallowing all kinds of waste and more quickly, However, that the material smells opens appetite, and thereby scientists game biotechnology those new hope in the possibility of restoring water corrections life cycle closed.

The Second World War was to come to an end even worked around the globe legend DDT to enter the world in the global war against many insect pests, insects and disadvantages of DDT began unfolding day after day in view of the firmness and high chemical solubility meager start accumulate in soil and water and slowly emerged adverse impacts on the various neighborhoods bringing one of the symbols of the failure of modern technology in harmony and harmony with nature circular logic—that this dilemma and found a surprising drop us coefficient of genetic engineering has been able team of researchers from the reprogramming of some strains of soil bacteria to introduce genes can produce the composite structure of a protein where permitted spatial molecule containing DDT inside cover and isolated from the environment to prevent influence-threatening environment.

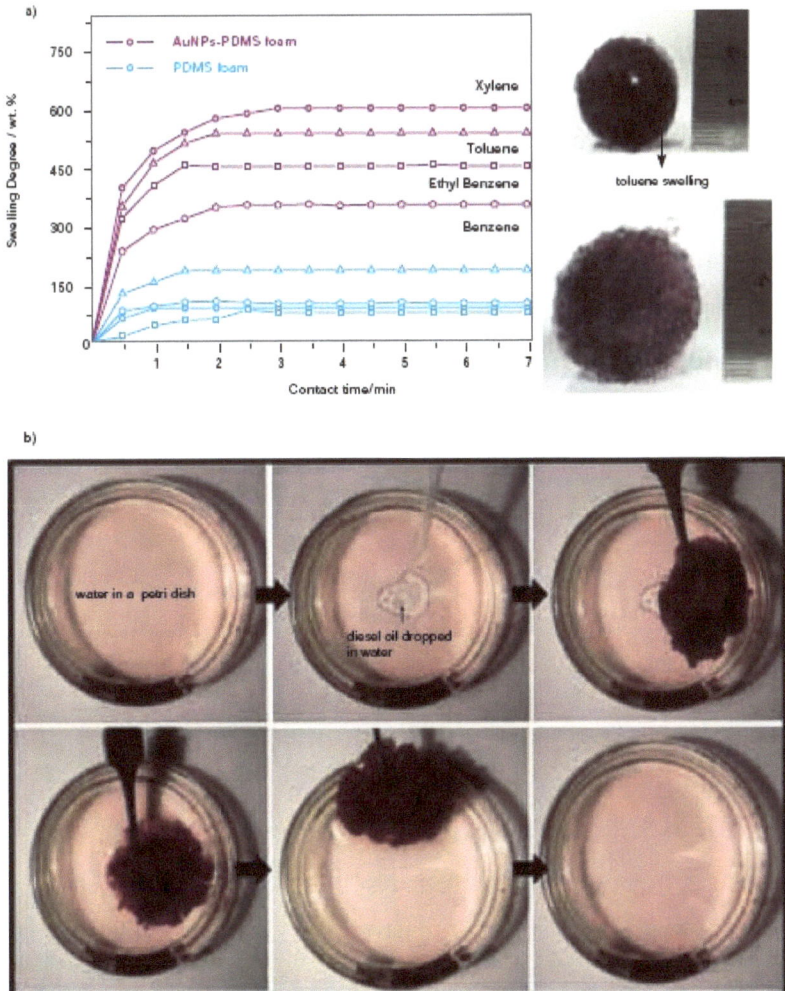

Removal of industrial organic pollutants (BTEX) and oil spills from water: (a) uptake curve for benzene, toluene, ethyl benzene and xylene present in contaminated water for PDMS and AuPDMS foams. (b) Demonstration for removal of diesel oil in water. Diesel uptake capacity of AuPDMS is 125% of its weight, and the uptake happens within minutes.

CHAPTER 9

Nitrogen Fertilizer

That there are millions of microorganisms in the soil capable of correcting the imbalance in the balance of nitrogen-the need for inorganic fertilizers. However, the usual rights hope to reap more food so feed more fertilizer plants, which in turn changed to some absorb nitrate plant to apply in his veins and the other part water leakage and every evil. What leakage of water has become a threat to fish but lost its validity for drinking water when the concentration of nitrates there. Let us image then and now what happens to humans when applied the nitrate in the digestive system.

There germs normal colon bacteria called disappoint deal with the transformation of nitrate to nitrite, which absorbs compound in the blood to interact with the hemoglobin levels prevent ability to transport oxygen, causing serious illness so-called (Methomogelopenemia), which causes the death of infants and natural disaster occur when vehicles nitrate soil under the influence of anaerobic bacteria since its conversion to Nitro and then to nitrogen oxides carbonated escalate into layers of the atmosphere, where the ozone layer, there is a slow erosion of this class of threats the entire life of that has scientists looking for a solution to restore the ecological balance was logical that these scientists is to develop new plant varieties have the ability to absorb nitrogen from the air directly or through bacterial strains repeat synthesis live with a living symbiotic which inevitably shatter for dispensing with fertilizer industrial, which represents a threat to the environment.

The Nitrogen Cycle is one of our planet's most vital nutrient or biogeochemical cycles because nitrogen is an essential building block of all the amino acids, which make up proteins, and is a critical element of the nucleic acids, DNA and RNA.

In short, without the nitrogen life as we know it is impossible.

There is no shortage of the element nitrogen here; it makes up 78-79% of our atmosphere. The atmosphere's nitrogen, N_2, has a very strong triple bond between the two atoms. Under normal conditions, it will not react with anything and either plants or animals cannot use it.

For plants to be able, to make use of the nitrogen they need the bond broken and recombined as either ammonia NH_3, NH_4 or nitrate NO_3. This process is called fixing or nitrogen fixation.

As plants need fixed nitrogen and we rely directly, either by eating plants or indirectly, by eating animals that have eaten plants, on them for our lives, fixed nitrogen is critical to life. Fixed or biologically available nitrogen is often the limiting factor for growth in an ecosystem or garden.

Bacteria handle the vast majority of the movement of fixed nitrogen. There is an intricate web of these bacteria in the soil. This diagram, compiled by USDA shows some of the flows of fixed and unfixed nitrogen in the soil.

Decomposer bacteria keep the fixed nitrogen in the system, Roughly, 1,200 million tons of fixed nitrogen is cycled back and forth through cycles of growth and decay in plants and animals because fixed nitrogen is often the limiting nutrient in an ecosystem nature carefully recycles this nutrient through the decomposers.

The composting process of decomposing is essentially the same thing-a way to breakdown the nutrients and keeps them an available in a plant friendly form.

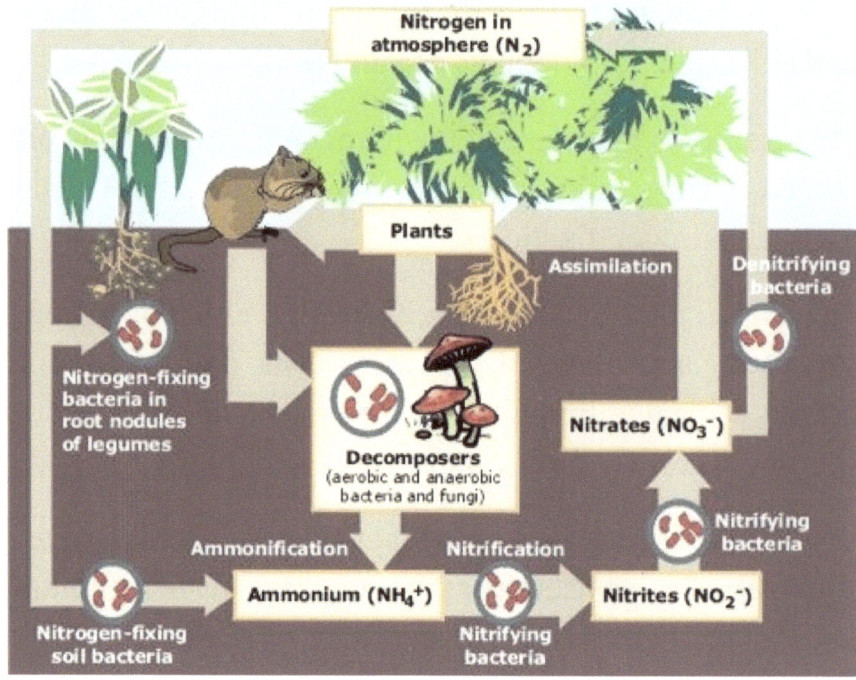

Another important group of bacteria denitrifies the fixed nitrogen releasing it back as N2 gas. The denitrifies keep the whole system in balance. Roughly, the same amount of nitrogen is fixed and then unfixed in the natural system.

These bacteria are vital to the life cycle of the planet. Many live in a symbiotic relationship with plants. The most well-known pairing are rhizobia bacteria with legumes plants. Indeed, agriculture's deliberate growing of legume crops contributes to some extent to the amount of nitrogen fixed throughout the year.

Another natural path for nitrogen fixing, one that is missing in the USDA diagram is that of lightning.

According to the National Severe Storms Laboratory, lightning can have between 100 million to a billion volts and contains billions of watts. It superheats the air to temperatures up to 60,000 degrees F in a matter of a few millionths of a second. This superheating produces very high pressures to develop (in fact; the pressure is what causes thunder).

The tremendous pressures and energy of a lightning flash are sufficient to break apart the triple nitrogen bond. The released atoms are then free to bond with the hydrogen and oxygen atoms in the water - rain - and they fall as mild nitrate and ammonium fertilizers.

While scientists argue about the extent of nitrogen fixed, it is worth noting that lightning strikes somewhere on the planet an average of 3 million times a day. Most scientists figure that 10 to 20 million tons of N are fixed this way. Likely, the first life forms relied on lightning as their source of the nitrogen building blocks.

Currently we, using an energy intensive process, now manage to fix around 100 million tons of nitrogen a year 80 million tons of which is used in fertilizer. This process developed by Fritz Haber in 1909 is an epic, which has had epic impacts on the planet.

CHAPTER 10

Oil Pollution

The environmental scientists in the world knew well CAUTION oil pollution, particularly maritime routes followed by oil tankers be concentrated along the continental shelf in waters off the coast, these are all areas of particular importance to the productivity of the sea, both staple food for marine organisms or products of various economic basic, as these areas are fisheries and traded with high importance, which represents a threat economically and environmentally inevitably now : what can scientists genetic engineering to eliminate the pollution of the sea oil? The truth is that there are many amazing ideas, and one of these ideas adopted by the American company General Electric, when enable researchers to create bacteria capable of engulfing the oil spilled in the waters of the seas and oceans have chosen scientists group three elements of the natural bacteria each with the capacity to devour any partial oil every part or one of the structure. Since the breeding grounds desired to develop bacteria capable of swallowing oil partly, but not a whole has spent in the work crossbreeding kinds of bacteria three minutes, painstaking work requiring vaccination of some or transplantation characteristics others and manipulates different genes. In addition, those actions resulted in a new bacterium does not exist in nature, and can swallow whole oil... The product active for some treatments for biotechnological problems of environmental pollution, both what has been accomplished buildings, which is expected to be completed during the next few years, hints clearly the success in some of these catch the treatments where the laws of nature did not overpowering clash, such treatments were forced to fractures and ruptures one of the flaws in the environmental life while so far failed treatments biotechnology which again find their way to closing sessions of the same environmental efficiency. Thus, the new environmental problems that might result in some of those new treatments than requires necessarily further reflection on the full and continued environmental audit, in the hope of achieving the principle of harmony and harmony with the logic of natural ecological cycles .. And anticipated results will depend on the extent of our understanding of the nature of environmental laws and respect, and that it is an integral whole that indivisible... and then being placed in this context, the need to test seriously each new step in the field of genetic engineering and testing of the interaction between each organism derived and environmental conditions in the labs before they enter natural environment.

The oil spills from oil tankers on land surface as well as in seas and oceans are a significant environmental hazard. This not only kills the aquatic flora and fauna by destroying the habitat but also creates health problems for the local inhabitants. Traditionally chemical dispersants are being used as remediation efforts. However, these chemical dispersants are also toxic in nature and they persist in the environment for a long time. The present techniques of washing the oil off the gravel and cleaning the area of oil spills, is very expensive and time consuming. In order to overcome some of these problems, the oleophilic fertilizers are being developed which allow rapid growth and multiplication of microbes, which further leads to the increase in the biodegradation process for removal of oil. In recent years, using genetic engineering, oil utilizing microorganisms have been produced which can grow rapidly on oil. The genetically engineered microbes for cleaning oil spills are mixed with straw. At the site of oil spill, the straw mixed with microbes are scattered over the oil-spilled area. The straw soaks the oily water and the microbes break the oil into non-toxic and non-polluting materials thereby cleaning up the site.

Some of the oil-utilizing microbes can also produce surface-active compounds that can emulsify oil in water and thereby remove the oil. A strain of *Pseudomonas aeruginosa* produces a glycolipid emulsifier that reduces the surface tension of oil-water interface, which helps in the removal of oil from water. This microbial emulsifier is nontoxic and biodegradable and has shown promising results in the laboratory experiments.

Some of the microorganisms, which are capable of degrading petroleum, include pseudomonads, various corynebacteria, mycobacteria and some yeast. The two methods for bioremediation of oil spills are a) using a consortium of bacteria and b) using genetically engineered bacteria/microbial strains.

 (Discussed under the topic of bioremediation) Both bacterial and fungal cultures from the petroleum sludge have been isolated.

 The fungal culture could degrade 0.4% sludge in 3 weeks. Degradation of petroleum sludge occurred within two weeks when the bacterial culture *(Bacillus circulars* CI) was used. A significant degradation of petroleum sludge was observed in 10 days when the fungus + *B. Circulars* and a prepared surfactant were exogenously added to petroleum sludge.

Based on a report published by the Society for Industrial Microbiology and tests performed by Bio-Aquatic of Pro-Act's Oil Clean bioremediation system — Oil Clean significantly outperforms all other bioremediation products.

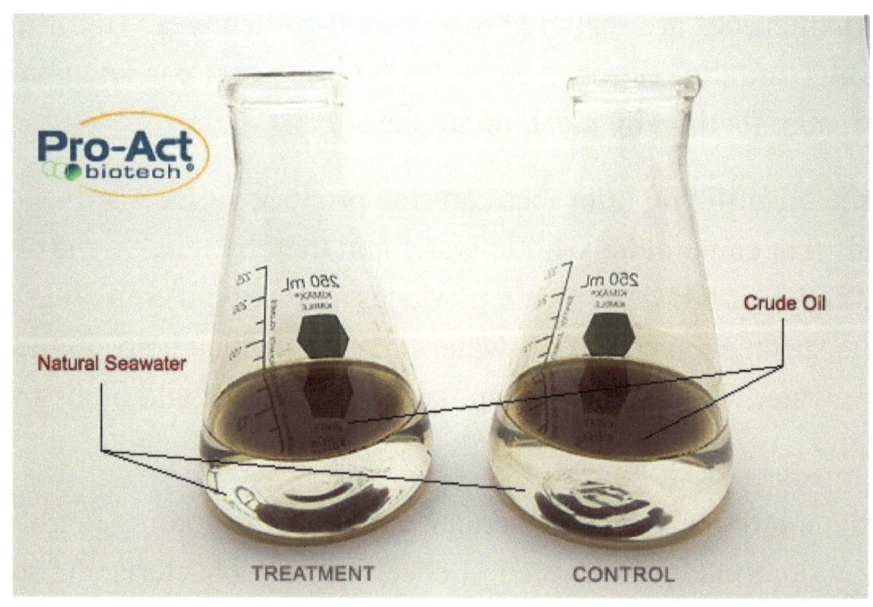

Two flasks were filled with equal amounts of seawater. Then equal amounts of crude oil were added to each flask.

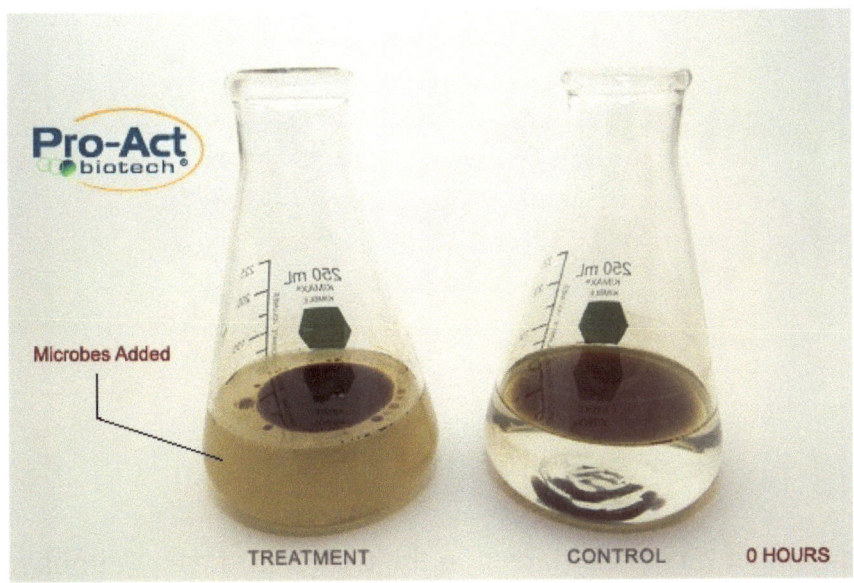

0 Hours

Our specialized eco-safe microbes and activator were added to the treatment flask (left). The control flask (right) was not altered. Both flasks were placed in an incubation unit (shaken to provide aeration). In an actual coastal or wetland habitat, aeration naturally occurs with tides, currents or external aerators.

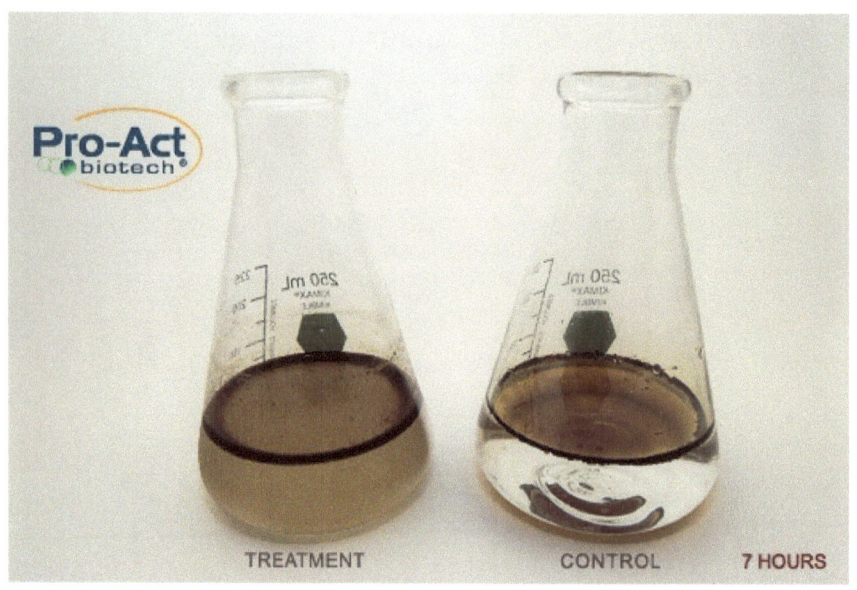

7 Hours

There is no longer an oil-like sheen in the treatment flask --, unlike control flask.

Microbes produce surfactants (similar to the chemical dispersant, but natural and safe to human, animals and the environment) that dissolved some crude oil in the water. The disappearance of crude oil on the water surface results as the oil particles fuse together and cling to the glass surface.

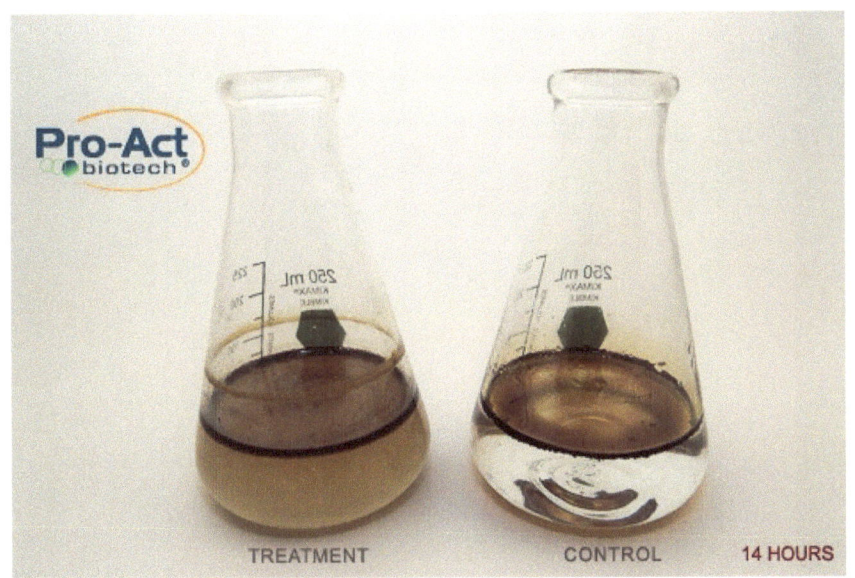

14 Hours

Seven hours later, the dark ring of oil is noticeably thinner in the treatment flask, as the microbes actively degrade the oil. The control flask remains the same.

As the degradation process continues, microbes are reproducing inside the flask. The speed of the degradation process depends on a number of factors such as temperature, nutrients, amount of dissolved oxygen present in the water and hydrocarbon chain length.

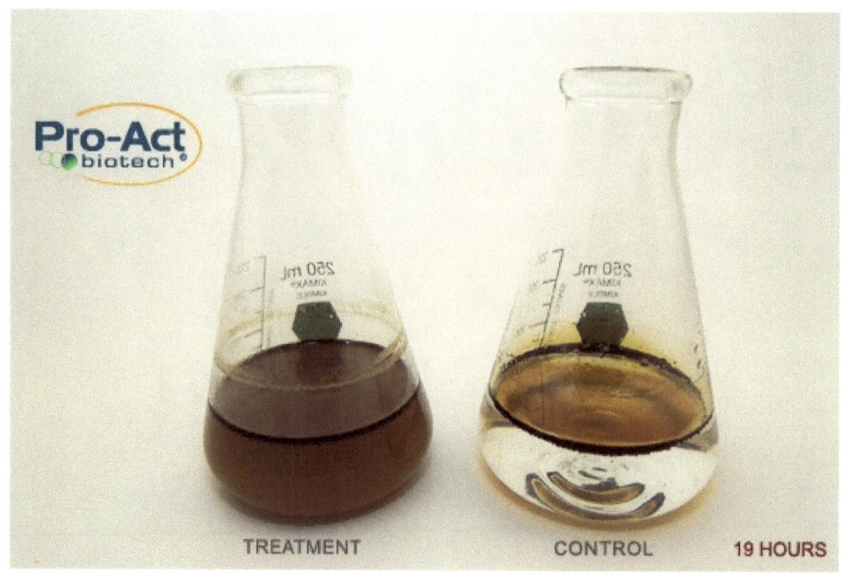

19 Hours

Five hours later, the dark ring of oil is diminishing in the treatment flask. The seawater is noticeably darker due to the breakdown and discernment of the oil in the presence of surfactants. This process is not harmful to ecosystems, unlike toxic chemical dispersants.

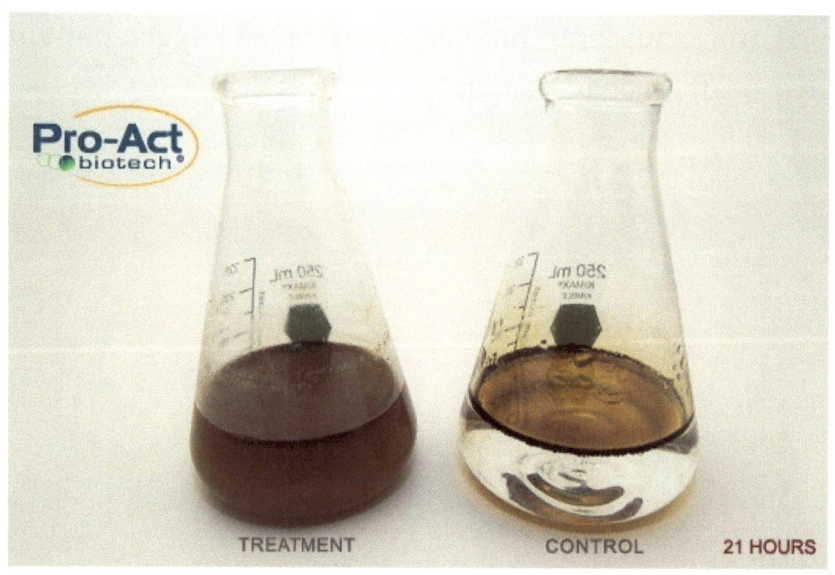

21 Hours
In less than a day of incubation, very little crude oil was visible in the treatment flask.

Not all-natural seawater is the same. There are many factors such as geological locations, tide and other conditions. Some oil degrading microbes exist in the Gulf water, but the number is relatively small. By augmenting oil degrading microbes, we can speed up the bioremediation process and help clean up the Gulf faster.

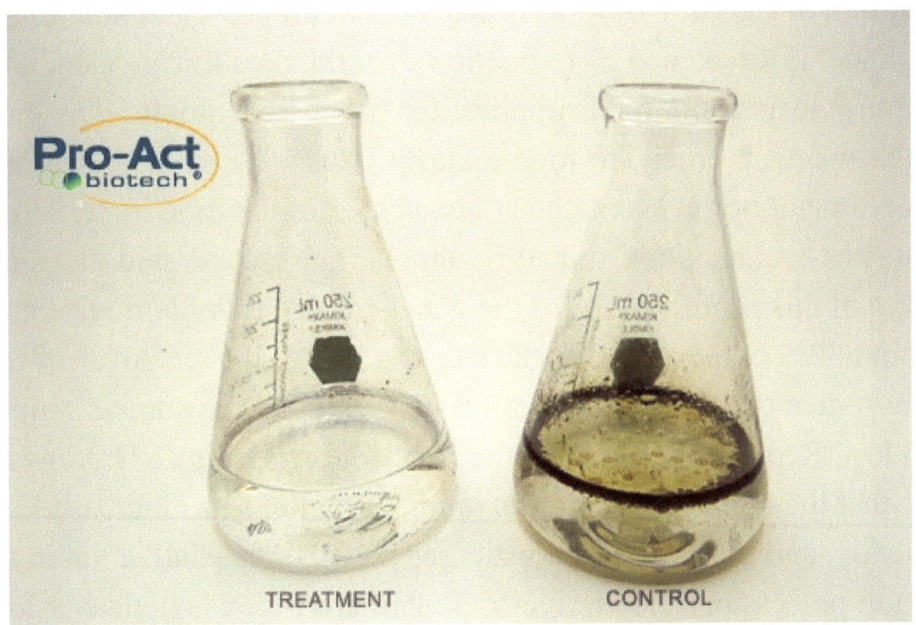

Treatment *(representation)*: After treatment with Oil Clean, the natural microbe-rich seawater will be dispersed with the flux of tides and weather, and digested by filter-feeding organisms such as crabs, shrimp and shellfish. The seawater will become decontaminated -- as it was before the oil disaster.

Without microbial treatment, the oil-devastated Gulf coast wetlands and marshes will endure for countless decades.

CHAPTER 11

Gene and Food

God created the earth in the balance calculated and furnished in natural resources necessary for life and has given biodiversity, which is the foundation for environmental safety and food security source and economic future generations is lifeline on Earth, but human sought during the past centuries to the welfare and prosperity at the expense of nature and balances breach draining its resources and reports indicate the Food and Agriculture Organization of the United Nations that 25% of all plant and animal species on this planet is threatened by extinction over the next thirty years, which will increase fears about food supplies for future generations. The plant genetic resources is crucial to food security especially since there are products of plant origin estimated at about 13% of the food material benefit of Rights has decided Food and Agriculture Organization said that since the beginning of this century, 75% of the genetic diversity of agriculture crops lost. About 30% of the earth's surface that is free of the ice cover of forests and forest when exposed to the erosion just removed the numbers more trees are also lost. Reports also indicate the Food and Agriculture Organization indicate that the rate of extinction of animal's factions has increased dramatically, and the reason in most cases is higher specialization in the production process of modern livestock. Perhaps Stock genetic erosion in general throughout the world are mostly economic reasons, social and political Consumption of genetic resources are increasingly part of a small and wealthy people in the world in terms of the devastating effects caused by poor people and its desperate struggle for survival on the other hand were two key to destroy the natural genetic sources. and genetic engineering has been characterized in that man for the first time in history has possessed the means to leverage underlying genetic stock in all organisms, whether plant, animal or micro-organisms including satisfy the ambitions of any crew that genetic or genotypes of the images of life can be different that placed on the table of genetic processes to be adapted to surgery for the development of genetic variations in genes known and is a natural result of the evolution of life. Because of environmental pollution, water shortages and lack of food and desertification all worries of world today.

Genetically engineered foods have had foreign genes (genes from other plants or animals) inserted into their genetic codes.

Selective breeding over time created these wide variations, but the process depended on the nature to produce the desired gene. Humans then chose to mate individual animals or plants that carried the particular gene in order to make the desired characteristics more common or more pronounced.

Genetic engineering allows scientists to speed this process up by moving desired genes from one plant into another -- or even from an animal to a plant or vice versa.

Some of the advantages of gene-modified foods:

The world population has topped 6 billion people and is predicted to double in the next 50 years. Ensuring an adequate food supply for this booming population is going to be a major challenge in the years to come. GM foods promise to meet this need in a number of ways:

☐ Pest resistance Crop losses from insect pests can be staggering, resulting in devastating financial loss for farmers and starvation in developing countries. Farmers typically use many tons of chemical pesticides annually.

Consumers do not wish to eat food that has been treated with pesticides because of potential health hazards, and run-off of agricultural wastes from excessive use of pesticides and fertilizers can poison the water supply and cause harm to the environment. Growing GM foods such as B.T. corn can help eliminate the application of chemical pesticides and reduce the cost of bringing a crop to market.

☐ Herbicide tolerance for some crops, it is not cost-effective to remove weeds by physical means such as tilling, so farmers will often spray large quantities of different herbicides (weed-killer) to destroy weeds, a time-consuming and expensive process that requires care so that the herbicide does not harm the crop plant or the environment. Crop plants genetically engineered to be resistant to one very powerful herbicide could help prevent environmental damage by reducing the amount of herbicides needed. For example, Monsanto has created a strain of soybeans genetically modified to be not affected by their herbicide product Roundup ®. A farmer grows these soybeans, which then only require one application of weed-killer instead of multiple applications, reducing production cost and limiting the dangers of agricultural waste run-off.

☐ Disease resistance there is many viruses, fungi and bacteria that cause plant diseases. Plant biologists are working to create plants with genetically engineered resistance to these diseases.

☐ Cold tolerance Unexpected frost can destroy sensitive seedlings. An antifreeze gene from cold-water fish has been introduced into plants such as tobacco and potato. With this antifreeze gene, these plants can tolerate cold temperatures that normally would kill unmodified seedlings.

☐ Drought tolerance/salinity tolerance as the world population grows, and more land is utilized for housing instead of food production, farmers will need to grow crops in locations previously unsuited for plant cultivation. Creating plants that can withstand long periods of drought or high salt content in soil and groundwater will help people to grow crops in formerly inhospitable places.

☐ Nutrition Malnutrition is common in third world countries where impoverished peoples rely on a single crop such as rice for the main staple of their diet. However, rice does not contain adequate amounts of all necessary nutrients to prevent malnutrition. If rice could be genetically engineered to contain additional vitamins and minerals, nutrient deficiencies could be alleviated. For example, blindness due to vitamin A deficiency is a common problem in third world countries. Researchers at the Swiss Federal Institute of Technology Institute for Plant Sciences have created a strain of "golden" rice containing an unusually high content of beta-carotene (vitamin A). Since the Rockefeller Foundation funded this rice, a non-profit organization, the Institute hopes to offer the golden rice seed free to any third world country that requests it. Plans were underway to develop golden rice that also has increased iron content.

However, the grant that funded the creation of these two rice strains was not renewed, perhaps because of the vigorous anti-GM food protesting in Europe, and so this nutritionally enhanced rice may not come to market at all.

☐ Pharmaceuticals Medicines and vaccines often are costly to produce and sometimes require special storage conditions not readily available in third world countries. Researchers are working to develop edible vaccines in tomatoes and potatoes. These vaccines will be much easier to ship, store and administer than traditional injectable vaccines.

☐ Phytoremediation Not all GM plants are grown as crops. Soil and groundwater pollution continues to be a problem in all parts of the world. Plants such as poplar trees have been genetically engineered to clean up heavy metal pollution from contaminated soil.

Potential risks include:

- Modified plants or animals may have genetic changes that are unexpected and harmful.

- Modified organisms may interbreed with natural organisms and out-compete them, leading to extinction of the original organism or to other unpredictable environmental effects.

- Plants may be less resistant to some pests and more susceptible to others.

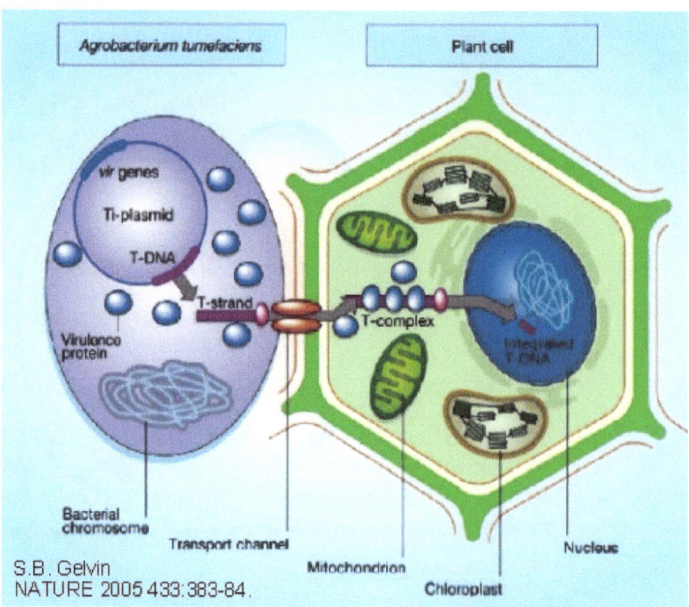

Agrobacterium tumefaction are commonly used in the genetic modification of plants

CHAPTER 12

Gene Bank

Many of our crops today are grown in massive fields around the world, and at times, these crops can be put at risk. For example, climate change might affect how crops grow in certain areas or introduce new pests. Disease and other natural or fabricated disasters also might destroy crops. To ensure that these crops are not permanently eradicated, species' researchers store the crops' genes in gene banks. It is also important that these researchers store the genes from different species of the same crop, such as the thousands of species of potatoes from around the world. That way, if something wipes out one species, a similar species can replace it. Scientists also can use the essential genetic information from various species of the plant to engineer a new, disease-resistant variety of that plant.

Single food crops can feed millions of people. There are about 7,000 crops that are used around the world to feed either people or animals, and there are millions of varieties of these thousands of crops [source: Government of the Netherlands]. Though that sounds like many crops, not every plant grows well in every region and climate, or under every circumstance. The land may not be as productive, and pests that used to stay away could find the new climate a friendly habitat and the crops a ready meal. Natural disasters, disease or human folly might wipe out entire harvests. Storing food crops' genes is a safeguard against any possible future disaster. Biodiversity also is critical to sustaining food for people and animals. If one plant becomes extinct, it might not seem important, but it can affect food chains and ecosystems.

Another reason scientist want to save plant genes in banks is to have them available for possibly breeding new varieties of crops that can better survive in a changing environment. If the climate continues warming, for example, crop species might have to adapt, and creating cultivars of plants that can better handle conditions created by climate change can ensure crop survival . There are about 1,500 gene banks located around the world to house crop material and provide a steady food supply in the event of natural disaster. Some of the banks have duplicate supplies of the same crops; this is by design so that if something happens to the supply at one bank, there is backup material at another.

The genetic sources of this and similar bank deposits and balances of the commercial banks.

It comprises four main sections bank namely: -1) the exploration and collection of genetic resources, this section based planning and implementation of exploratory missions to locate a genetic source then collected is receiving genetic sources of genetic other banks. 2) Processing Section textures and crews genetic The Section processing genotypes through isolate genetic material DNA or gene undesirable or chromosomal gene carriers can also be processed in other ways genotypes differ by source type genotype For example in the case of plant genetic resources can be saved or group of cells plant tissue that can evolve under conditions that are suitable for growth to give new plants, seeds or other plant parts as part of the leg, suggested some plant cells, in the case of nitrogen and microbial genetic resources can be conserved in private farms containing glycerol means nitrogen. 3) Section multiplication and evaluation: -and has a crew of genetic propagation and follow-up. 4) The documentation section: - registering and maintaining information on bank balances of genetic sources with computers to facilitate information with other gene banks and facilitate the utilization of genetic resources in collaboration with institutions and scientific institutes specialized.

The genotypes and crews distinct genetic cornerstone programs in genetic engineering and genetic sources contained in plant, animal and microbial.

Gene banks store genetic material from plants or animals such as seeds, spores or eggs frozen in cold chambers at minus 20 degrees Celsius, keeping it intact for over 100 years for later use.

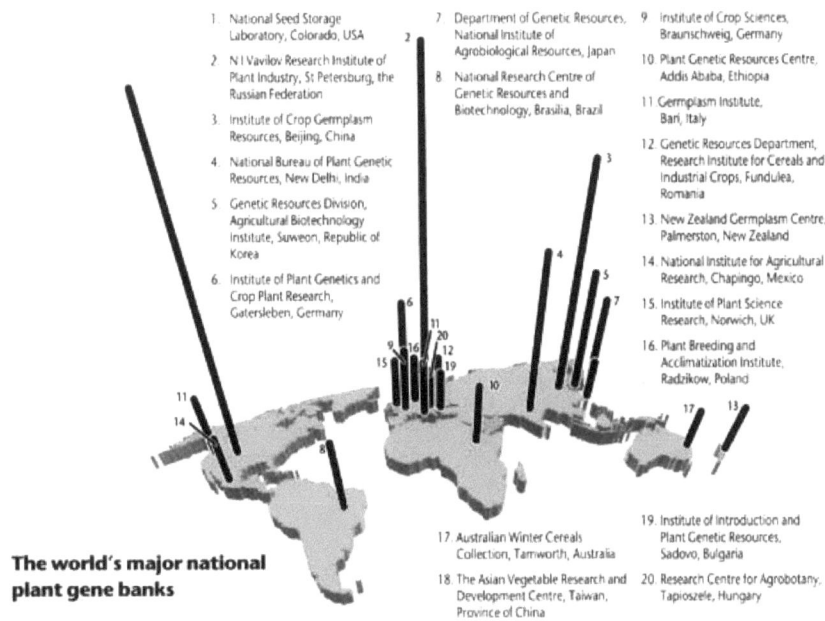

1. National Seed Storage Laboratory, Colorado, USA

2. N I Vavilov Research Institute of Plant Industry, St Petersburg, the Russian Federation

3. Institute of Crop Germplasm Resources, Beijing, China

4. National Bureau of Plant Genetic Resources, New Delhi, India

5. Genetic Resources Division, Agricultural Biotechnology Institute, Suweon, Republic of Korea

6. Institute of Plant Genetics and Crop Plant Research, Gatersleben, Germany

7. Department of Genetic Resources, National Institute of Agrobiological Resources, Japan

8. National Research Centre of Genetic Resources and Biotechnology, Brasília, Brazil

9. Institute of Crop Sciences, Braunschweig, Germany

10. Plant Genetic Resources Centre, Addis Ababa, Ethiopia

11. Germplasm Institute, Bari, Italy

12. Genetic Resources Department, Research Institute for Cereals and Industrial Crops, Fundulea, Romania

13. New Zealand Germplasm Centre, Palmerston, New Zealand

14. National Institute for Agricultural Research, Chapingo, Mexico

15. Institute of Plant Science Research, Norwich, UK

16. Plant Breeding and Acclimatization Institute, Radzikow, Poland

The world's major national plant gene banks

17. Australian Winter Cereals Collection, Tamworth, Australia

18. The Asian Vegetable Research and Development Centre, Taiwan, Province of China

19. Institute of Introduction and Plant Genetic Resources, Sadovo, Bulgaria

20. Research Centre for Agrobotany, Tapioszele, Hungary

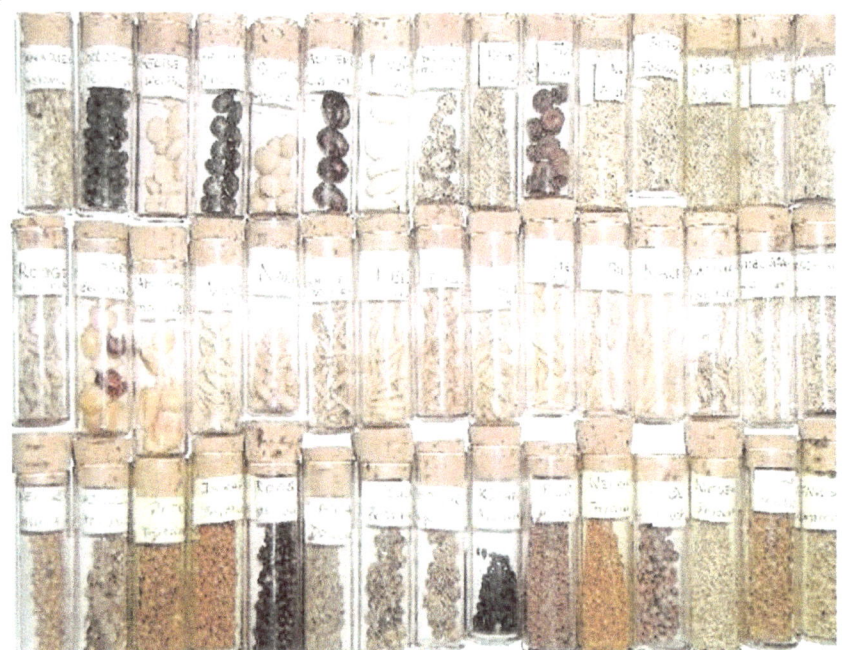

Gene Bank

CHAPTER 13

Cloning Vital

The term cloning describes a number of different processes that can be used to produce genetically identical copies of a biological entity. The copied material, which has the same genetic makeup as the original, is referred to as a clone.

Researchers have cloned a wide range of biological materials, including genes, cells, tissues and even entire organisms, such as a sheep.

In nature, some plants and single-celled organisms, such as bacteria, produce genetically identical offspring through a process called asexual reproduction. In asexual reproduction, a new individual is generated from a copy of a single cell from the parent organism.

Natural clones, also known as identical twins, occur in humans and other mammals. These twins are produced when a fertilized egg splits, creating two or more embryos that carry almost identical DNA. Identical twins have nearly the same genetic makeup as each other, but they are genetically different from either parent.

There are three different types of artificial cloning: gene cloning, reproductive cloning and therapeutic cloning.

Gene cloning provides copies of genes or segments of DNA. Reproductive cloning provides copies of whole animals. Therapeutic cloning produces embryonic stem cells for experiments aimed at creating tissues to replace injured or diseased tissues.

Gene cloning, also known as DNA cloning, is a very different process from reproductive and therapeutic cloning. Reproductive and therapeutic cloning shares many of the same techniques, but is done for different purposes.

Researchers routinely use cloning techniques to make copies of genes that they wish to study. The procedure consists of inserting a gene from one organism, often referred to as "foreign DNA," into the genetic material of a carrier called a vector. Examples of vectors include bacteria, yeast cells, viruses or plasmids, which are small DNA circles carried by bacteria. After the gene is inserted, the vector is placed in laboratory conditions that prompt it to multiply, resulting in the gene being copied many times over.

In reproductive cloning, researchers remove a mature somatic cell, such as a skin cell, from an animal that they wish to copy. They then transfer the DNA of the donor animal's somatic cell into an egg cell, or oocyte that has had its DNA-containing nucleus removed.

Researchers can add the DNA from the somatic cell to the empty egg in two different ways. In the first method, they remove the DNA-containing nucleus of a somatic cell with a needle and inject it into an empty egg. In the second approach, they use an electrical current to fuse the entire somatic cell with the empty egg.

In both processes, the egg is allowed to develop into an early-stage embryo in the test-tube and then is implanted into the womb of an adult female animal. Ultimately, the adult female gives birth to an animal that has the same genetic makeup as the animal that donated the somatic cell. This young animal is referred to as a clone. Reproductive cloning may require the use of a surrogate mother to allow development of the cloned embryo, as was the case for the most famous cloned organism, Dolly the sheep.

Over the last 50 years, scientists have conducted cloning experiments in a wide range of animals using a variety of techniques. In 1979, researchers produced the first genetically identical mice by splitting mouse embryos in a test tube and then implanted the resulting embryos into the wombs of adult female mice. Shortly after that, researchers produced the first genetically identical cows, sheep and chickens by transferring the nucleus of a cell taken from an early embryo into an egg that had been emptied of its nucleus.

It was not until 1996, however, that researchers succeeded in cloning the first mammal from a mature (somatic) cell taken from an adult animal. After 276 attempts, Scottish researchers finally produced Dolly, the lamb from the udder cell of a 6-year-old sheep. Two years later, researchers in Japan cloned eight calves from a single cow, but only four survived.

Besides cattle and sheep, other mammals that have been cloned from somatic cells include cat, deer, dog, horse, mule, ox, rabbit and rat. In addition, a rhesus monkey has been cloned by embryo splitting.

Despite several highly publicized claims, human cloning still appears to be fiction. There currently is no solid scientific evidence that anyone has cloned human embryos.

In 1998, scientists in South Korea claimed to have successfully cloned a human embryo, but said the experiment was interrupted very early when the clone was just a group of four cells. In 2002, cloned is part of a religious group that believes humans were created by extraterrestrials, held a news conference to announce the birth of what it claimed to be the first cloned human, a girl named Eve. However, despite repeated requests by the research community and the news media, Clonaid never provided any evidence to confirm the existence of this clone or the other 12 human clones it purportedly created.

In 2004, a group led by Woo-Suk Hwang of Seoul National University in South Korea published an article in the journal *Science* in which it claimed to have created a cloned human embryo in a test tube. However, an independent scientific committee later found no proof to support the claim and, in January 2006, *Science* announced that Hwang's paper had been retracted.

From a technical perspective, cloning humans and other primates is more difficult than in other mammals. One reason is that two proteins essential to cell division, known as spindle proteins, are located very close to the chromosomes in primate eggs. Consequently, removal of the egg's nucleus to make room for the donor nucleus also removes the spindle proteins, interfering with cell division. In other mammals, such as cats, rabbits and mice, the two spindle proteins are spread throughout the egg. Therefore, removal of the egg's nucleus does not result in loss of spindle proteins. In addition, some dyes and the ultraviolet light used to remove the egg's nucleus can damage the primate cell and prevent it from growing.

Reproductive cloning may enable researchers to make copies of animals with the potential benefits for the fields of medicine and agriculture.

For instance, the same Scottish researchers who cloned Dolly have cloned other sheep that have been genetically modified to produce milk that contains a human protein essential for blood clotting. The hope is that someday this protein can be purified from the milk and given to humans whose blood does not clot properly. Another possible use of cloned animals is for testing new drugs and treatment strategies. The great advantage of using cloned animals for drug testing is that they are all genetically identical, which means their responses to the drugs should be uniform rather than variable as seen in animals with different genetic make-ups.

After consulting with many independent scientists and experts in cloning, the U.S. Food and Drug Administration (FDA) decided in January 2008 that meat and milk from cloned animals, such as cattle, pigs and goats, are as safe as those from non-cloned animals are. The FDA action means that researchers are now free to using cloning methods to make copies of animals with desirable agricultural traits, such as high milk production or lean meat. However, because cloning is still very expensive, it will likely take many years until food products from cloned animals appear in supermarkets.

Another application is to create clones to build populations of endangered, or possibly even extinct, species of animals. In 2001, researchers produced the first clone of an endangered species: a kind of Asian ox known as a guar. sadly, the baby guar, which had developed inside a surrogate cow mother, died just a few days after its birth. In 2003, another endangered type of ox, called the Banteg, was successfully cloned. Soon after, three African wildcats were cloned using frozen embryos as a source of DNA. Although some experts think cloning can save many species that would otherwise disappear, others argue that cloning produces a population of genetically identical individuals that lack the genetic variability necessary for species' survival.

Some people also have expressed interest in having their deceased pets cloned in the hope of getting a similar animal to replace the dead one.

However, as shown by Cc the cloned cat, a clone may not turnout exactly like the original pet whose DNA was used to make a clone.

Reproductive cloning is a very inefficient technique, and most cloned animal embryos cannot develop into healthy individuals. For instance, Dolly was the only clone to be born live out of 277 cloned embryos. This very low efficiency, combined with safety concerns, presents a serious obstacle to the application of reproductive cloning.

Researchers have observed some adverse health effects in sheep and other mammals that have been cloned. These include an increase in birth size and a variety of defects in vital organs, such as the liver, brain and heart. Other consequences include premature aging and problems with the immune system. Another potential problem centers on the relative age of the cloned cells chromosomes. As cells go through their normal rounds of division, the tips of the chromosomes, called telomeres, shrink. Over time, the telomeres become so short that the cell can no longer divide and, consequently, the cell dies.

 This is part of the natural aging process that seems to happen in all cell types. Therefore, clones created from a cell taken from an adult might have chromosomes that are already shorter than normal, which may condemn the clones' cells to a shorter life span. Indeed, Dolly, who was cloned from the cell of a 6-year-old sheep, had chromosomes that were shorter than those of other sheep were her age. Dolly died when she was six years old, about half the average sheep's 12-year lifespan.

Therapeutic cloning involves creating a cloned embryo for the sole purpose of producing embryonic stem cells with the same DNA as the donor cell. These stem cells can be used in experiments aimed at understanding disease and developing new treatments for disease. To date, there is no evidence that human embryos have been produced for therapeutic cloning.

The richest source of embryonic stem cells is tissue formed during the first five days after the egg has started to divide. At this stage of development, called a blastocyst, the embryo consists of a cluster of about 100 cells that can become any cell type. Stem cells are harvested from cloned embryos at this stage of development, resulting in the destruction of the embryo while it is still in the test tube.

Researchers hope to use embryonic stem cells, which have the unique ability to generate virtually all types of cells in an organism, to grow healthy tissues in the laboratory that can be used replace injured or diseased tissues.

In addition, it may be possible to learn more about the molecular causes of disease by studying embryonic stem cell lines from cloned embryos derived from the cells of animals or humans with different diseases. Finally, differentiated tissues derived from ES cells are excellent tools to test new therapeutic drugs.

Many researchers think it is worthwhile to explore the use of embryonic stem cells as a path for treating human diseases. However, some experts are concerned about the striking similarities between stem cells and cancer cells. Both cell types can proliferate indefinitely, and some studies show that after 60 cycles of cell division, stem cells can accumulate mutations that could lead to cancer. Therefore, the relationship between stem cells and cancer cells needs to be more clearly understood if stem cells are to be used to treat human disease.

Gene cloning is a carefully regulated technique that is broadly accepted today and used routinely in many labs worldwide. However, both reproductive and therapeutic cloning raises important ethical issues, especially as related to the potential use of these techniques in humans.

Reproductive cloning would present the potential of creating a human that is genetically identical to another person who has previously existed or who still exists.

This may conflict with long-standing religious and societal values about human dignity, possibly infringing upon principles of individual freedom, identity and autonomy. However, some argue that reproductive cloning could help sterile couples fulfill their dream of parenthood. Others see human cloning as a way to avoid passing on a deleterious gene that runs in the family without having to undergo embryo screening or embryo selection.

Therapeutic cloning, while offering the potential for treating humans suffering from disease or injury, would require the destruction of human embryos in a test tube. Consequently, opponents argue that using this technique to collect embryonic stem cells is wrong, regardless of whether such cells are used to benefit sick or injured people.

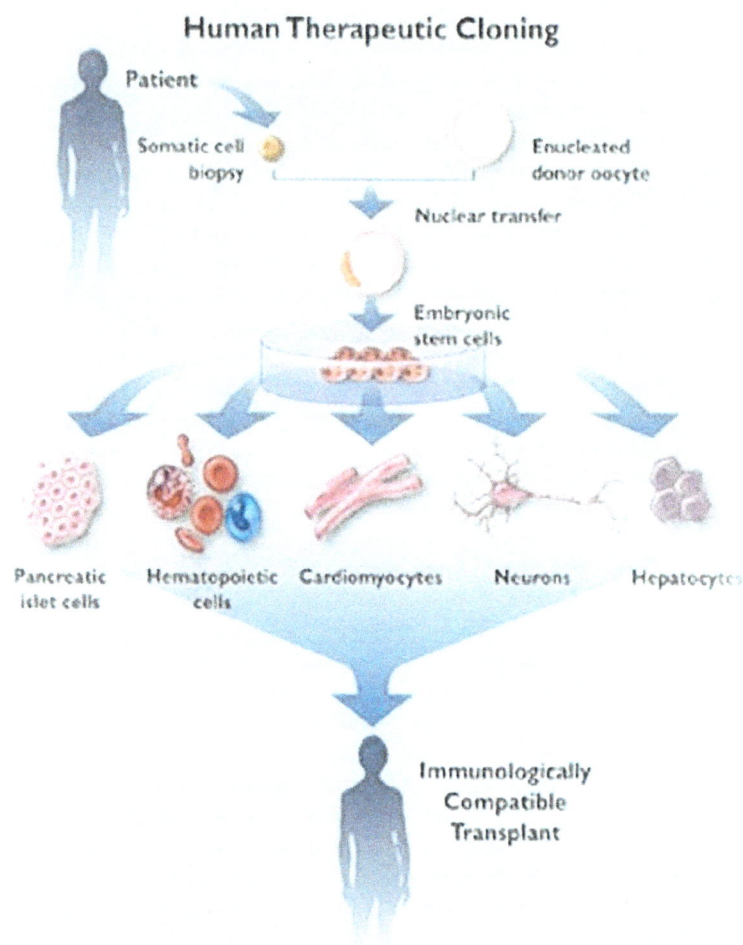

Advanced Cell Technology, Inc.,
Worcester, Massachusetts.

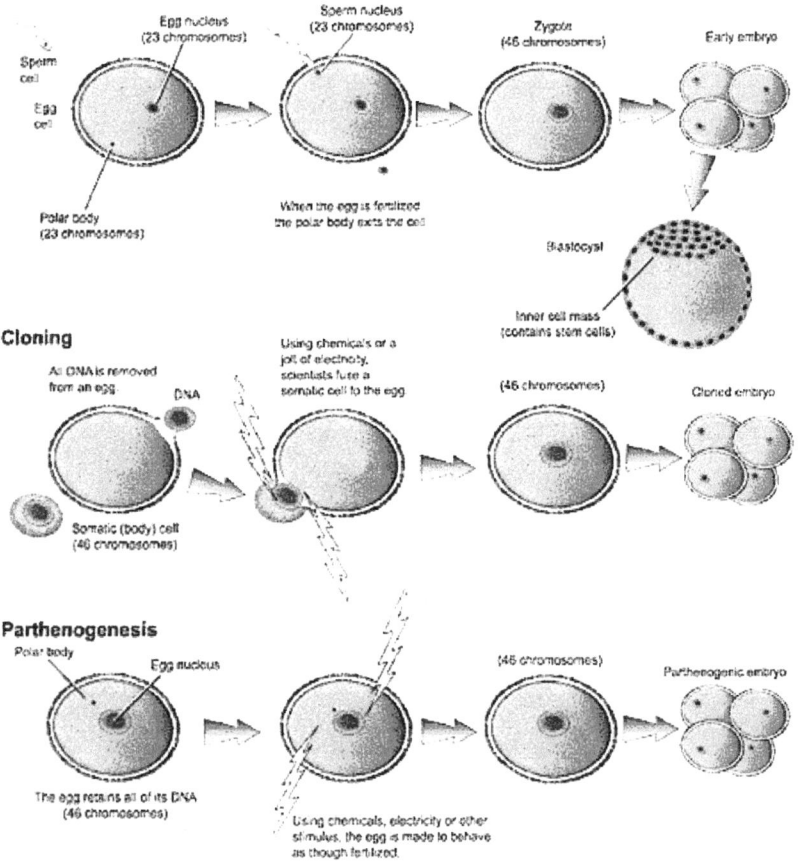

Diagram of early stages of human fertilization, cloning, and parthenogenesis.

[Modified from Rick Weiss and Patterson Clark, *The Washington Post*.]

CHAPTER 14

Immunology and AIDS

The science of immunology independent not only emerge in the 1950s and 1960s when technological development has enabled the identification of anatomical and functional structures of the immune system and show the uniqueness of lymph tissue function commander and coordinator of the immune defense operations.

During the 1980s the worldwide scientific and medical community struggled to understand the nature of the disease, to track down the human immunodeficiency virus (HIV) responsible for it, and to develop rudimentary treatments an effort that continued throughout the 1990s.

In the meantime, AIDS has continued to destroy lives.

The Joint United Nations Programmed on HIV/AIDS (UNAIDS) estimates that 36.1 million individuals around the world were living with HIV infections or full-blown AIDS at the end of last year.

In 2000 alone HIV/AIDS caused the deaths of approximately 3 million individuals, making a cumulative death toll of 21.8 million by year's end. UNAIDS' figures also indicate that roughly one in every 100 adults between the ages of 15 and 49 is now infected with HIV. More than 80 percent of all adult HIV infections have resulted from heterosexual intercourse.

Throughout the past decade the scientific and medical communities have sought better understanding of the HIV virus in hopes of developing more effective therapies, possibly including vaccines for individuals not exposed to the virus and for AIDS patients. Policy makers realize that they have a long road to travel before they begin to think about having this disease in check. "You not only. But also have the effect of the virus infecting the cell," says Anthony Fauci, director of the National Institute of Allergy and Infectious Diseases (NIAID). "The HIV envelope itself is an extraordinary entity in its ability to have an aberrant effect on the immune system. In addition to being a disease of immune deficiency, it is a disease of aberrant immune system activations. These effects are quite profound. Unfortunately for the human species HIV/AIDS is proving to be an extraordinary experiment of nature about its effects on the immune system."

The result of AIDS knows detailed (acquired Immune Deficiency Syndrome) from obstructed labor human immunodeficiency virus HIV in the central cells of the immune system and destroy these cells called T4 assistance or CD4, which are like the orchestra leader for the Immune coordinate and harmonize between the different immune responses leading to the erosion of the census, these cells gradually to Landing immunological function of the patient is ultimately phase Immune Deficiency respiratory and becomes susceptible to various infections, tumors and has provided innovative techniques scientists accurately on the life cycle of HIV testing is conducted on patients infected with the possible use of antiretroviral drugs for HIV estimate half-life of the virus and the rapid propagation and compensation were found to be HIV take occasional invasion of the cell while generating new viral particles to invade other cells about 2.6 day also estimated the number of viral particles generated daily in these patients by about ten billion viral molecule any rate multiplication of the virus and destroy cells and the high-end over an extended period, but what does that mean? How can these facts be a source of optimism?

 In fact, it further if the defense forces capable of achieving balance with the virus and keep it under control for a period of more than ten years, despite the use of the virus through all this period has spent the reproduction and development, we can upset the balance in favor of final a strong immune and one of two ways : strengthening defenses the body and makes it more ability to produce effective responses to the HIV virus is weakening or make it more vulnerable to these forces, or a combination of both cross Maybe we had to change the mentality that we were dealing with this factor in contravention of the nurse now we have become accustomed during our dealings with other infectious diseases.

The researchers will soon have achieved many important discoveries that could have a significant impact on future strategies, especially in the area of prevention and treatment has finally been disclosed, "Assistant acceptant" to secure the entry of the virus into the cell and modification has been known for a long time that the CD4 located on the surface of T4 is contact with HIV surface protein, but this association was not enough to invade the cell and start life cycle for an extended period of occupancy this acceptant ready to entry process for scientists around the world that was discovered recently by a research team from the National Institute of sensitivity and infectious diseases in the "Bethesda" state of Maryland. Named acceptant new (FUSION) that this acceptant is a vehicle similar play the same role in different cells for different viral strains.

There is no doubt that this evolutionary surge will continue, AIDS virus is still with us even more dangerous alleviation There is still room for original contributions and creative, which is needed more than ever to join a global scientific effort to rid humanity of the plague of the twentieth century.

Researchers and clinicians working in multidisciplinary teams have made steady progress in countering the virus. For example, the research effort that isolated the HIV virus and then sequenced and cloned its various genes to express its proteins led about a decade ago to protease inhibitors. "This class of drugs has been shown to be extraordinarily efficient when used with other drugs," says Fauci. "To me this is a classic example of the translation from basic research to clinical benefit."

Drug cocktails containing protease inhibitors have significantly extended the lives of many patients. In addition, the search for other active forms of chemical therapy continues. "What we would like to see from a new class of drugs is the same impact as protease inhibitors," says Richard Colon, vice president of infectious disease discovery at pharmaceutical company Bristol-Myers Squibb. "We see similar inhibition levels with the new class of entry inhibitors. New drugs will give patients an expanded set of options for combining drugs and avoiding long-term toxicity."

Behavioral concepts have also proved valuable for individual patients. For example, interrupted therapy permits individual patients to take occasional breaks from their drug regimens, giving them some relief from the often-devastating side effects that those regimens cause.

A team at the Lifespan/Tufts/Brown Center for AIDS Research (CFAR) is refining a project that pays neighbors to deliver AIDS treatments to patients who have difficulty reaching a hospital or doctor's office for therapy. "So far we've achieved results in terms of reducing viral loads far better than before," says Charles Carpenter, committee chair of CFAR and professor of medicine at Brown University. "We're also looking at nutrition. In women, the body-mass index correlates positively with the length of time before the patient gets serious symptoms after being infected."

All those approaches lack one essential element. While they slow down the progress of HIV infection or full-blown AIDS, they do not result in a reconstitution of HIV-specific immunity. Therefore, the search is on for a vaccine — or perhaps several vaccines — that will confer at least some immunity to the virus. Vaccines can be used in an attempt to prevent initial infection or to slow progression of the disease if a person becomes infected despite having been vaccinated. In addition, vaccine trials have been initiated in people who are already infected in an attempt to boost HIV-specific immunity.

To date approximately 30 vaccines against HIV have been tested, most in phase 1 or phase 2 trials to determine their safety and immunogenicity. Only one vaccine candidate, made by VaxGen, Inc., has gone on to phase 3 efficacy trials, which will probably not be completed for some time. Development of an HIV vaccine has become a very high priority in AIDS research. The National Institutes of Health expects to spend $282 million on research into vaccines this year, one-eighth of its entire AIDS budget. Several pharmaceutical companies have also entered the arena.

Within the past few months, the effort has started to show definite promise. "Vaccines provide another example of how in-the-trenches basic research is showing us the light at the end of the tunnel that was very dark for a long time," says Fauci. "Right now we feel certainly more optimistic than we felt a year ago about the possibility of developing an HIV vaccine."

The research has application beyond AIDS. "The natural experiment of HIV is teaching us more about the human immune system than many decades of animal research," says Fauci. "HIV has, in a grossly horrific way, given us clues to how the immune system works," echoes Chow.

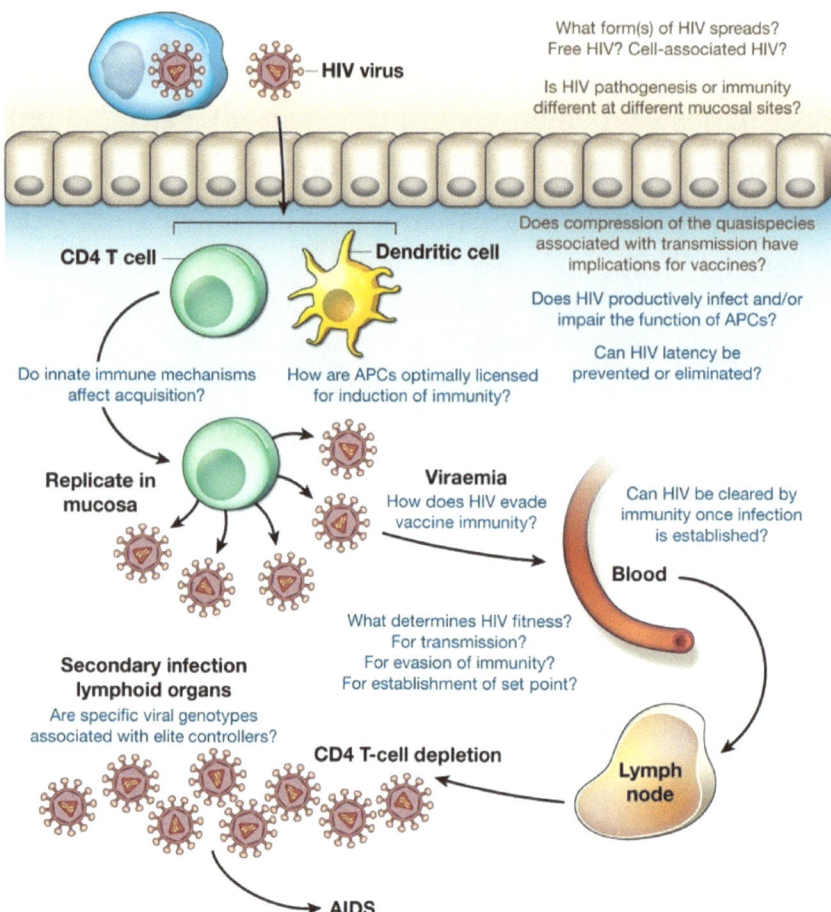

CHAPTER 15

Diagnosis of Viral Diseases

In general, diagnostic tests can be grouped into three categories:

(1) Direct detection, (2) indirect examination (virus isolation), and (3) serology.

In direct examination, the clinical specimen is examined directly for the presence of virus particles, virus antigen or viral nucleic acids. In indirect examination, the specimen into cell culture, eggs or animals in an attempt to grow the virus: this is called virus isolation. Serology constitutes by far the bulk of the work of any virology laboratory. A serological diagnosis can be made by the detection of rising titers of antibody between acute and convalescent stages of infection, or the detection of IgM. In general, the majority of common viral infections can be diagnosed by serology. The specimen used for direction detection and virus isolation is critical. A positive result from the site of disease would be of much greater diagnostic significance than those from other sites.

For example, in the case of herpes simplex encephalitis, a positive result from the CSF or the brain would be much greater significance than a positive result from an oral ulcer, since reactivation of oral herpes is common during times of stress.

1. Direct Examination of Specimen

 1. Electron Microscopy morphology / immune electron microscopy

 2. Light microscopy histological appearance - e.g. inclusion bodies

 3. Antigen detection immunofluorescence, ELISA etc.

 4. Molecular techniques for the direct detection of viral genomes

2. Indirect Examination

1. Cell Culture - cytopathic effect, haemadsorption, confirmation by neutralization, interference, immunofluorescence, etc.

2. Eggs pocks on CAM - haemagglutination, inclusion bodies

3. Animals disease or death confirmation by neutralization

3. Serology

Detection of rising titers of antibody between acute and convalescent stages of infection, or the detection of IgM in primary infection.

Reliable diagnosis some viral diseases like influenza, measles and parotid gland on the patient's clinical symptoms, which show a clear, but some other diseases such as inflammation hepatitis and AIDS, the AIDS laboratory diagnosis, diagnosis is a necessity in this situation is by isolating the virus and identify it is a difficult issue requiring specialized labs a high level of processing and possibilities laboratory and trained human being or through diagnosis to confirm the existence of antibodies formed in the patient's blood to attack the virus and attempt to rid the body of knowledge and quantity analysis or radio-immunoassay kit.

Because of the difficulty of growing viruses in cell cultures living lab or diagnosed by conventional means scientists have tended to use genetic engineering methods to detect viruses in the samples directly without turning to follow through segregation rules in the viral DNA known as a test enzyme polymerization reactions (PCR), the serial is important This test reveals that the least amount of the virus in the sample and thus the diagnosis of infection can occur at the beginning and is an important step in the early diagnosis of viral infection before the appearance of symptoms.

 For example, the crossing in the case of infection with hepatitis C distinct anti-virus composed after infection and continues during directly for a very long time even after recovery; in addition to that of the PCR test can determine the type of virus strain.

The example reflects the importance of this is that it so far has been the discovery of five strains of HIV hepatitis C are not responding to treatment by interferon usual, thanks to identify race before treatment begins to be very costly addition to the side effects that no longer on the patient recovery. It is thus clear that the PCR test shows the picture before attending the physician, which helped select the ideal method of treatment.

Significant technical advances have occurred, especially in the last five years, in the laboratory diagnosis of viral infections.

Immunologic detection of immediate early antigens in specimens such as bronchoalveolar lavage fluid and blood inoculated into shell via cell cultures, particularly for herpes virus (cytomegalovirus, herpes simplex virus, varicella-zoster virus), has presented results 16 to 48 hours after inoculation rather than the several days required for recognition of cytopathic effects in conventional tube cell cultures. Similarly, cytomegalovirus viremia can be detected directly by immunostaining of peripheral blood leukocytes with commercially available reagents the same day the specimen is submitted to the laboratory. Single-test membrane immunoassays have provided rapid (15 minutes) detection of viral antigens (respiratory syncytial virus, rotavirus, influenza virus type A). In the near future, diagnostic virology laboratories will be expected to monitor viral strains for susceptibility to the growing list of antiviral drugs. Amplification of nucleic acid sequences of viruses from cerebrospinal fluid or tissue, which does not yield isolated by conventional diagnostic techniques, has added a new dimension to the laboratory diagnosis of viral infection.

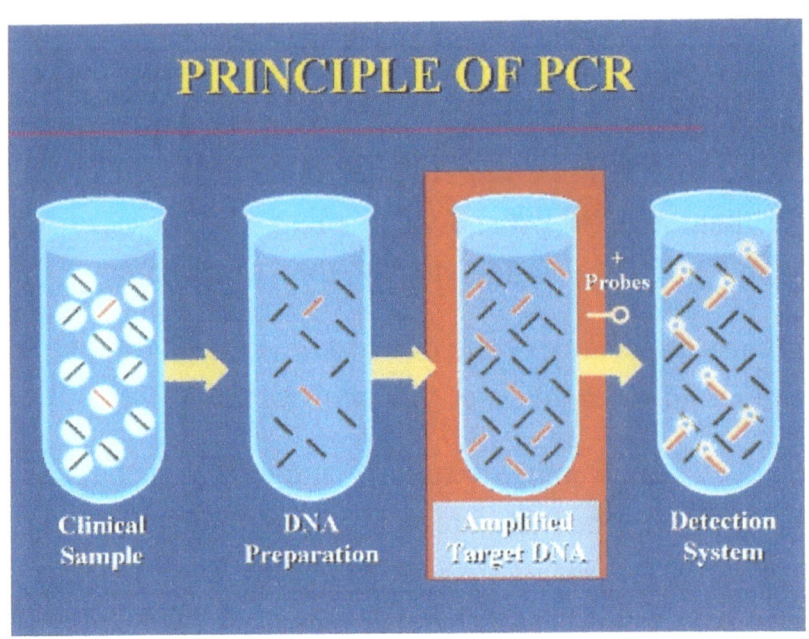

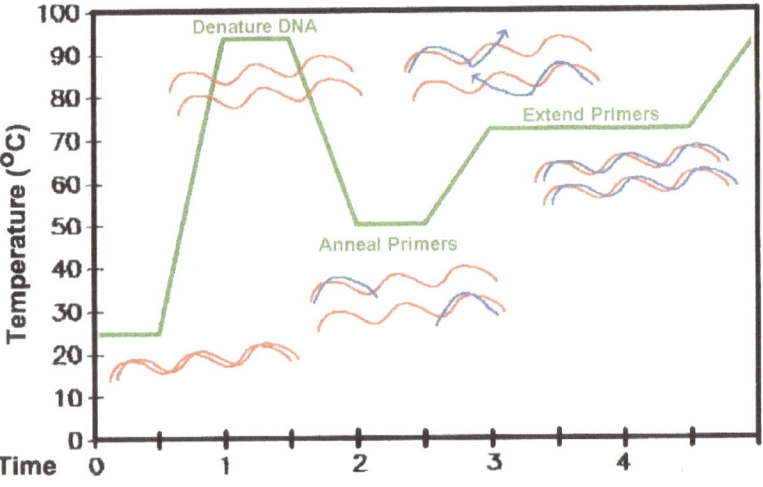

The Polymerase Chain Reaction (PCR)

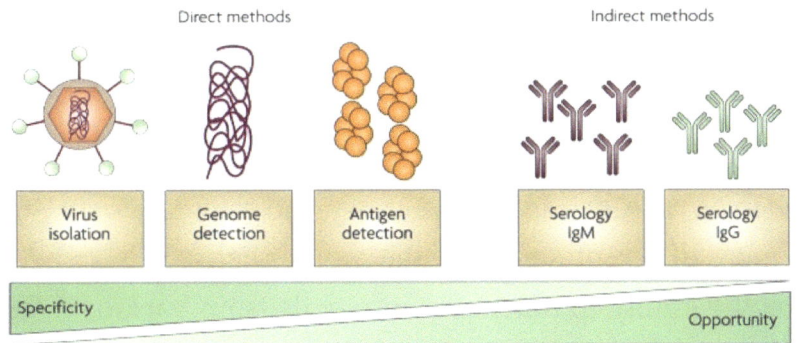

Direct and indirect diagnostic tests for dengue

CHAPTER 16

Stem Cells

Stem cells (SCs) are characterized by self-renewability, i.e. the ability to divide themselves rapidly and continuously and to create new SCs and progenitors more differentiated than the mother cells. SCs show high plasticity, i.e. the ability to transform into cells from various different tissues. The plasticity can be explained by trans-differentiation (direct or indirect) and fusion. Trans-differentiation is the acquisition of the identity of a different phenotype through the expression of the gene pattern of another tissue. By fusion with a cell of another tissue, an SC can express a gene from that cell and acquire a phenotypic element of another tissue.

In the human body, adult stem cells (ASCs) maintain the tissue homeostasis. ASCs, usually, differentiate in a restricted range (multi-potent) of progenitors and terminal cells to replace old and damaged cells.

SCs derived from early human embryos (Embryonic stem cells (ESCs)), on the other hand, are plural-potent and can generate all committed cell types. Fetal stem cells (FSCs) derive from the placenta, membranes, amniotic fluid or fetal tissues.

Since the use of embryonic and fetal stem cells is highly restricted and not without risk due to the potential induction of malignant tumors, the following review focuses on the properties and clinical applications on adult human stem cells (AHSC).

Time-lapse imaging and tracking of single human embryonic stem cells has allowed researchers to zoom in and take a closer look at the behavior of these specialized cells.

Researchers from the University of Sheffield have identified multiple bottlenecks that restrict the growth of these cells in the laboratory, and observed complex and diverse behavior as the cells move around the culture dish and interact with their neighbors.

These findings will help researchers design the best conditions safely and efficiently to grow human embryonic stem cells in the laboratory.

Numerous clinical trials have attempted to test the benefits of using a patient's stem cells (taken from the bone marrow) to treat heart disease. Results have been conflicting; some claim significant improvements in heart function, whilst others report none at all. A group at Imperial College London investigated the possible reasons for this inconsistency and found strange, unexplained discrepancies within reports of many of the clinical trials. They have identified a link between claimed success rates and discrepancies, casting doubts over the validity of this treatment.

- 133 reports of 49 clinical trials were investigated
- 600+ discrepancies were found
- Discrepancies ranged from minor to serious mistakes and misrepresentation of data
- Reports with the most discrepancies claimed most benefit to patients, while those without discrepancies showed no improvement in patients' conditions.

Researchers at the Hebrew University of Jerusalem have developed a new cocktail that is highly effective at coaxing adult cells to become quality pluripotent stem cells.

Regenerative medicine is a new and expanding area that aims to replace lost or damaged cells, tissues or organs through cellular transplantation. Because stem cells derived from human embryos can trigger ethical concerns, a good solution is reprogramming adult cells back to an embryo-like state using a combination of reprogramming factors.

The resulting cells, called induced pluripotent stem cells (iPSCs), could be used to replace those lost to damage or disease. However, scientists have discovered that the process of reprogramming adult cells can introduce genetic abnormalities that limit the cells' usefulness in research and medicine.

To make iPSCs, scientists expose adult cells to a cocktail of genes that are active in embryonic stem cells. iPSCs can then be coaxed to differentiate into other cell types such as nerve or muscle. However, the standard combination of factors used to reprogram cells leads to a high percentage of serious genomic aberrations in the resulting cells. (The reprogramming factors are Oct4, Sox2, Klf4, and Myc - known collectively as OSKM).

Now researchers at the Hebrew University of Jerusalem have developed a new cocktail of reprogramming factors that produce high-quality iPSCs. Dr. Youssef Buganim, at the Institute for Medical Research Israel-Canada in the Hebrew University's Faculty of Medicine, worked with scientists at the lab of Whitehead Institute founding member Rudolf Jaenisch, a professor of biology at MIT.

The researchers reasoned that changing the reprogramming factors could reprogram the adult cells in a more controlled way and yield high-quality iPSCs. Working with mouse cells, Dr. Buganim and research scientist Styling Markoulaki used bioinformatics analysis to design a new cocktail of reprogramming factors (Sall4, Nano, Err, and Lin28, known collectively as SNEL).

Their results showed that the interaction between reprogramming factors plays a crucial role in determining the quantity and quality of resulting iPSCs - and that a different combination of reprogramming factors can in fact produce a much higher quality product.

The new SNEL cocktail created fewer colonies of iPSCs, but approximately 80% of those produced passed the most stringent pluripotency test.

This is highly preferable to the traditional OSKM cocktail, which produces a large number of colonies, but the majority of which fail the pluripotency test.

Dr. Buganim hypothesizes that SNEL may reprogram cells better than OSKM because it does not rely on the master regulators Oct4 and Sox2, which might activate part of the adult cell genome. According to Buganim, the research demonstrates the effectiveness of bioinformatics tools in producing high-quality iPSCs.

This study takes the regenerative medicine field one-step closer to the clinic, where it may be able to help patients in need of cellular transplantation therapy. The researchers will now seek to define the optimal combinations for reprogramming human iPSCs, which are harder to reprogram than mouse cells and which could not be reprogrammed using the SNEL cocktail.

University of British Columbia, in collaboration with Beta Logics Venture, a division of Janssen Research & Development, LLC, has published a study highlighting a protocol to convert stem cells into insulin-producing cells. The new procedure could be an important step in the fight against Type 1 diabetes.

The protocol can turn stem cells into reliable, insulin-producing cells in about six weeks, far quicker than the four months it took using previous methods.

"We are a step closer to having an unlimited supply of insulin-producing cells to treat patients with Type 1 diabetes," says Timothy Kieffer, who led the research and was a professor in UBC's Department of Cellular and Physiological Sciences and the Department of Surgery.

The protocol transforms stem cells into insulin-secreting pancreatic cells via a cell-culture method. The conversion is completed after the cells are transplanted into a host.

"We have not yet made fully functional cells in a dish, but we are very close," says Kieffer. "The cells we make in the lab produce insulin, but are still immature and need the transplant host to complete the transformation into fully functioning cells."

An important next step for UBC researchers and their industry collaborators is to determine how to prevent the insulin-producing cells' from being rejected by the body. (The research was published in the journal *Nature Biotechnology*).

Using human induced pluripotent stem cells (hiPSCs), researchers have gained new insight into what may cause schizophrenia by revealing the altered patterns of neuronal signaling associated with this disease.

They did so by exposing neurons derived from the hiPSCs of healthy individuals and of patients with schizophrenia to potassium chloride, which triggered these stem cells to release neurotransmitters, such as dopamine, that are crucial for brain function and are linked to various disorders.

By discovering a simple method for stimulating hiPSCs to release neurotransmitters, the findings in the International Society for Stem Cell Research's journal *Stem Cell Reports*, published by Cell Press, could provide new insights into how neurons communicate with each other and could lead to a better understanding of the neural mechanisms underlying a range of brain disorders.

"This study is novel because it shows that stem cell neurons derived from patients can provide new insight into neurotransmitter mechanisms occurring in brain disorders such as schizophrenia," says senior study author Vivian Hook of the University of California, San Diego.

"The approach of this study has broad opportunities for uncovering the neurochemistry of brain cell communication in numerous brain disorders, via these studies of human disease in a dish. Findings from these studies will lead to new therapeutic strategies for brain disorders, especially those mental and neurological diseases for which no drug treatments exist today."

HiPSCS are cells that are taken from adults, genetically reprogrammed to an embryonic stem cell-like state, and then converted into specialized cells such as neurons. Patient-derived hiPSCs offer the possibility of modeling an individual's disease in a dish and assessing which drugs will most effectively treat the disease. Because dysfunction in neural communication is linked to brain disorders such as schizophrenia, Hook and Fred Gage of The Salk Institute and Kristen Brennand of the Icahn School of Medicine at Mount Sinai set out to determine whether hiPSC-derived neurons can be induced to release important brain signaling chemicals, allowing disease mechanisms to be studied in a dish.

To address this question, the researchers exposed hiPSC-derived neurons from healthy individuals and patients with schizophrenia to a chemical known to stimulate the release of neurotransmitters. They found that these cells contained neurotransmitter-producing enzymes and were capable of secreting dopamine, norepinephrine, and epinephrine - neurotransmitters that are crucial for brain function and that are linked to various disorders. Moreover, secretion of the three neurotransmitters was enhanced in hiPSC-derived neurons from schizophrenia patients compared with those from healthy individuals.

"The significance of this study is that patient-derived stem cell neurons can uncover previously unknown neurotransmitter brain mechanisms occurring in schizophrenia," Hook says," Because in vivo human brain research is limited, hiPSC neurons derived from patients create new opportunities to understand changes occurring in brain cells occurring in nervous system disorders. These approaches can potentially define new drug targets for the development of therapeutic agents to improve the lives of schizophrenia patients."

As we age, stem cells throughout our bodies gradually lose their capacity to repair damage, even from ordinary wear and tear. Researchers from the Ottawa Hospital Research Institute and University of Ottawa have discovered the reason this decline occurs in our skeletal muscle. Their findings were published online in the influential journal *Nature Medicine*.

A team led by Dr. Michael Rudnicki, senior scientist at the Ottawa Hospital Research Institute and professor of medicine at the University of Ottawa, found that as muscle stem cells age, their reduced function is a result of a progressive increase in the activation of a particular signaling pathway. Such pathways transmit information to a cell from the surrounding tissue. The particular culprit identified by Dr. Rudnicki and his team is called the JAK/STAT signaling pathway.

"What's really exciting to our team is that when we used specific drugs to inhibit the JAK/STAT pathway, the muscle stem cells in old animals behaved the same as those found in young animals," said Dr. Michael Rudnicki, a world leader in muscle stem cell research. "These inhibitors increased the older animals' ability to repair injured muscle and to build new tissue."

What is happening is that our skeletal muscle stem cells are not being instructed to maintain their population.

To maintain a population of these stem cells, which are called satellite cells, some have to stay as stem cells when they divide. With increased activity of the JAK/STAT pathway, fewer divide to produce two satellite cells (symmetric division) and more commit to cells that eventually become muscle fiber.

This reduces the population of these regenerating satellite cells, which results in a reduced capacity to repair and rebuild muscle tissue.

While this discovery is still at early stages, Dr. Rudnick's team is exploring the therapeutic possibilities of drugs to treat muscle-wasting diseases such as muscular dystrophy. The drugs used in this study are commonly used for chemotherapy, so Dr. Rudnicki is now looking for less toxic molecules that would have the same effect.

A team of researchers from Korea and Canada have found that transplantation of B10 cells (a stable immortalized human bone marrow-derived mesenchymal stem cell line; B10 has) directly into the bladder wall of mice modeled with spinal cord injury (SCI) helped inhibit the development of bladder fibrosis and improved bladder function by promoting the growth of smooth muscle cells in the bladder.

The study will be published in a future issue of *Cell Transplantation* and is currently freely available on-line as an unedited early e-pub.

Spinal cord injury (SCI) can cause severe lower urinary tract dysfunction and conditions such as overactive bladder, urinary retention and increased bladder thickness and fibrosis. HMSCs, multipotent cells that can differentiate into a variety of cell types, including bone cells, cartilage cells, and fat cells, have been transplanted into injured spinal cords to help patients regain motor function.

In this study, mice receiving the B10 hMSCs injected directly into the bladder wall experienced improved bladder function while an untreated control group did not.

"Human MSCs can secrete growth factors," said study co-author Seung U. Kim of the Division of Neurology at the University Of British Columbia Hospital, Vancouver, Canada. "In a previous study, we showed that B 10 cells secrete various growth factors including hepatocyte growth factor (HGF) and that HGF inhibits collagen deposits in bladder outlet obstructions in rats more than hMSCs alone. In this study, the SCI control group that did not receive B10 cells showed degenerated spinal neurons and did not recover. The B10-injected group appeared to have regenerated bladder smooth muscle cells."

Four weeks after the onset of SCI, the treatment group received the B10 cells transplanted directly into the bladder wall. To track the transplanted B10 cells via magnetic resonance imaging (MRI), the researchers labeled them with fluorescent magnetic particles.

"HGF plays an essential role in tissue regeneration and angiogenesis and acts as a potent antifibrotic agent," explained Kim.

The researchers concluded that the local injection, rather than systemic intravenous injection, was preferred because systemic injection caused the hMSCs to be localized in the pulmonary capillary bed.

Voiding function was assessed at four weeks post-transplantation and MRI "showed clear hypo intense signal induced by the labeled cells". When the bladders of the transplanted group were harvested, they were found to have improved smooth muscle cells and reduced collagen deposition.

The researchers concluded that MSC-based cell transplantation might be a novel therapeutic strategy for bladder dysfunction in patients with SCI.

"This study provides potential evidence that a human stable immortalized MSC line could be useful in the treatment of spinal cord injury-related problems such as bladder dysfunction.," said Dr. David Eve, associate editor of Cell Transplantation and Instructor at the Center of Excellence for Aging & Brain Repair at the University of South Florida.

"Further studies to elucidate the mechanisms of action and the long-term effects of the cells, as well as confirm the optimal route of administration, will help to illuminate what the actual benefit of these cells could be."

Thanks to significant discoveries in basic and clinical research and technological advances, the fight against cancer has mobilized into an elaborate offensive spanning multiple fronts.

Work happening in the University of Alberta chemistry lab could help new and more selective therapies for cancer. Researchers have developed a compound that targets a specific enzyme overexpressed in certain cancers - and they have tested its activity in cells from brain tumors.

Chemistry professor Christopher Cairo and his team synthesized a first-of-its-kind inhibitor that prevents the activity of an enzyme called neuraminidase. Although flu viruses use enzymes with the same mechanism as part of the process of infection, human cells use their forms of the enzyme in many biological processes.

Cairo's group collaborated with a group in Milan, Italy, that has shown that neuraminidases are found in excess amounts in glioblastoma cells, a form of brain cancer.

In a new study, a team from the University of Milan tested Cairo's enzyme inhibitor and found that it turned glioblastoma cancer stem cells - found within a tumor and believed to drive cancer growth - into normal cells. The compound also caused the cells to stop growing, suggesting that this mechanism could be important for therapeutics. Results of their efforts were published in the Nature journal *Cell Death & Disease.*

Cairo said these findings establish that an inhibitor of this enzyme could work therapeutically and should open the door for future research.

"This is the first proof-of-concept showing a selective neuraminidase inhibitor can have a real effect in human cancer cells," he said. "It isn't a drug yet, but it establishes a new target that we think can be used for creating new, more selective drugs."

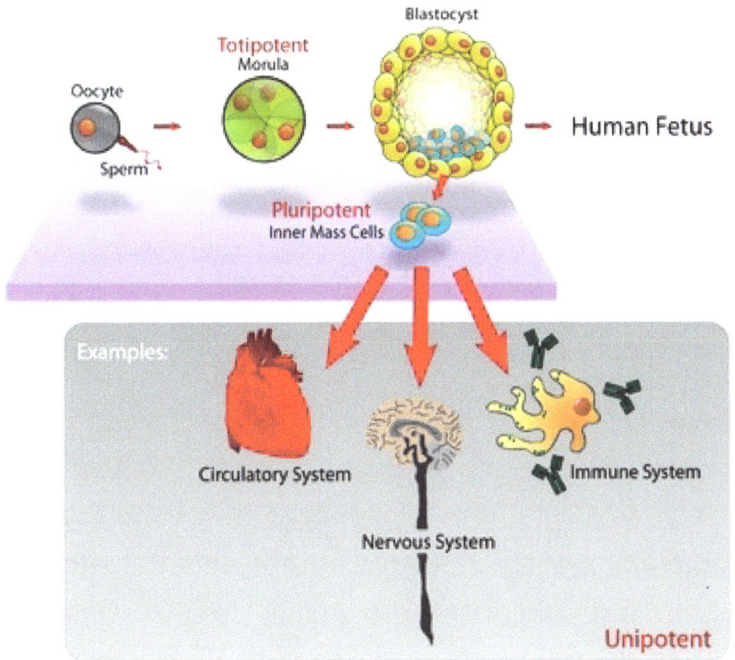

Wikipedia, stem cell, Main article: Cell potency

Pluripotent, embryonic stem cells originate as inner cell mass (ICM) cells within a blastocyst. These stem cells can become any tissue in the body, excluding a placenta. Only cells from an earlier stage of the embryo, known as the morula, are totipotent, able to become all tissues in the body and the extra embryonic placenta.

Targeting cancer stem cells to cure cancer ?

- Unlimited self-renewal
- Exclusive tumorigenicity
- Recapitulation of entire tumor
- **Resistance to standard therapy**

Tumor size / Days

Prior to chemotherapy   Chemotherapy   Chemotherapy

S.C&C Group

Eliminating the root of the tumors – Cancer stem cells are highly resistant to chemo-/radiotherapy and are assumed to represent the source of relapse. Targeted elimination of cancer stems cells should eventually lead to eradication of the tumor if combined with chemo-/radiotherapy.

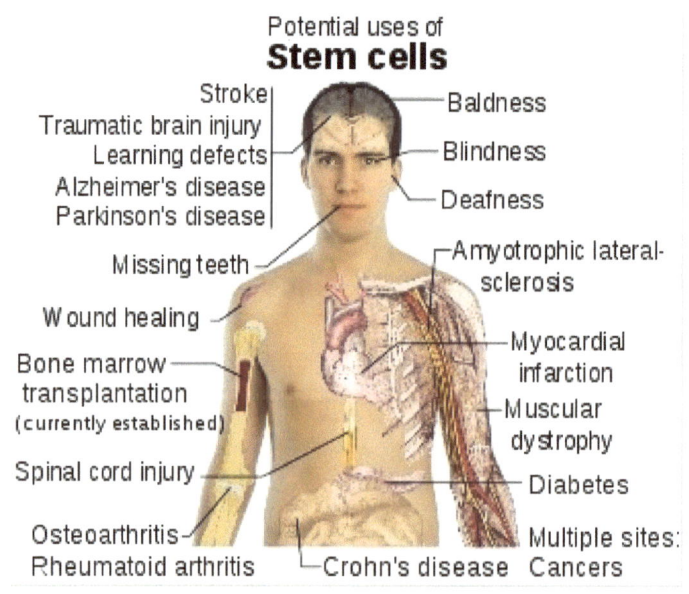

Potential uses of
Stem cells

Stroke
Traumatic brain injury
Learning defects
Alzheimer's disease
Parkinson's disease

Baldness
Blindness
Deafness

Missing teeth

Amyotrophic lateral-sclerosis

Wound healing

Bone marrow transplantation
(currently established)

Myocardial infarction
Muscular dystrophy

Spinal cord injury

Diabetes

Osteoarthritis
Rheumatoid arthritis

Crohn's disease

Multiple sites:
Cancers

Wikipedia, Examiner.com

Conclusion:

The great achievements in the field of biotechnological already served to deepen our understanding of the factors influencing the march of development and operations, especially those that have a significant impact in the evolution of the human race, people now know that some forms of advanced technology in the field of medicine and biological sciences were already available and could be used already and can be exploited in gene control as a lot of machines and technology complex, which brings us to the future, which allows us more room for governing gene widely after this, let alone the means available to us now that can be developed mainly If books for humans to open new areas wider Bioethics It is the secret of development it can then increase the speed of evolutionary process or to modify the way in which it wishes.

The scientists have consistently stressed that the progress of mankind depends on the progress of science free hand search, but they quickly for the laboratories and devised us artificial distinction between science and the results, after what appeared visible risk imposed on the path of science and misdeeds of applications that resulted in either the biggest proof of the weakness of feature neutrality in contemporary science, it is the pressure that surround it in the present day, the path taken by the flag meant originally that option was available to move in this way without this, but make science take the road means that there is a specific point of what it wanted to walk in the knowledge that point without the other.

It is not in the course of science inevitable or that it is impossible to put an end to it, because it is quite possible through the monitoring of the budget for scientific research admiration, but the point here that the financial budget of fun for science cannot be free from ideological considerations example, or particular values or preferences self wants to learn that much compared to the money that is spent. Whatever it is the factor of funding and spending on scientific research is only one side of the issue-the issue of neutrality in science-an external factor is the pressure on the face of science and nature from abroad, but there is another factor is the internal responsibility of scientists and researchers about future developments in the fields of science The impact on human progress, or delay.

References:

1-Brandenburg, Oliver. (INTRODUCTION TO MOLECULAR BIOLOGY AND GENETIC ENGINEERING), food and agriculture organization of the united nations, Rome, 2011.

2-Johnson, Dr.George, (GENE TECHNOLOGY), txtwriter Inc.

Three-(GENE TECHNOLOGY), commonwealth scientific and industrial research organization, 24 Jun 2010, updated/06 December 2013.

4-GENE TECHNOLOGY), the Merck Manual Home, Edition, August2013by David N.Finegold, MD.

5-(GENETICS HOME REFERENCE), service of the USA library of medicine, published September 15, 2014.

6-Mats Hansen, project leader of (Tasquinimod), (Active Biotech), Sweden.

7-(Gene Therapy Consortium), Tay-Sachs, 2007.

8-Wikimedia Commons, (Tay - Sachs disease), Encyclopedia.com

9-Fraunhofer Institute for Interfacial Engineering and Biotechnology, (Removing pollutants and contaminants from wastewater), Jul 26, 2013.

10-NicolaisL, Lavorgna M, (The biotechnology for removal of specific pollutants), PubMed ID: 12619386.

11-(Biotechnology in Environmental Monitoring and pollution abatement), Bio-Med Research international, Vol.2014, and Article ID: 235472.

12-Machadesch, Barbara, (Bacteria and biotechnology can clean up PHL water pollution, University of Philippines, January 19, 2012.

13-T.Nicholl, Desmond S., (An introduction to genetic engineering), Cambridge University, 3rd Edition.

14-(Biotechnology and Environment), Treatment of sewage using microorganisms, Biotechnology 4U, copyright2014.

15-(Genetic Testing During Pregnancy), Kids Health From Nemours.

16-(Centers for Disease Control and Prevention), Genomic Testing, USA.

17-National Cancer Institute, (Genes in the news), the national institutes of health.

18-Shahrokh F, Shariat, MD and Kevin M slawin, MD. (Reviews in Urology), PMCID: PMC1476102.

19-RS Ahima. (Obesity gene therapy: slimming immature rats), Gene therapy (2002)10,196-197, doi:10,1038/sj.gt.3301920,nature.com

19-Helene Choquet and David Meyre, (Genetics of Obesity: what have we learned?), PMCID: PMC 3137002.

20-El-Sayed Mustafa JS, Froquel P., (From Obesity genetics to the future of personalized obesity therapy), PMID: 23529041.

21-National Heart, Lung, and Blood Institute, (Working group report on future research directions in childhood obesity prevention and treatment), August 21-22, 2007.

22-American Heart Association, (Circulation Research), molecular medicine, Jun 25, 2004, Vol94 NO.121579-1588.

23-School of Medicine and Public Health, (Gene therapy for type 1 diabetes aims to eliminate daily insulin injections), 07/22/2013.

24-University of North Carolina school of medicine, (New gene therapy proves promising as hemophilia treatment), Science Daily, December 10, 2013.

25-National Heart, Lung, and Blood institute. (How is hemophilia treated), Jul 31, 2013.

26-Hemophilia-information.com., provided by Home Care for the Cure, (Cure for Hemophilia).

27-Mark Skinner. (Gene therapy for hemophilia: Addressing the coming challenges of Affordability and accessibility), Molecular Therapy (2013), 21 1,1-2,doi:10,1038/mt.2012,272,nature.com

27-American Society of Gene&Cell Therapy. (Type 1 Diabetes), 200-2011.

28-N Welsh., Gene Therapy,(Prospects for gene therapy of diabetes mellitus), *Department of Medical Cell Biology, Uppsala University, S-751 23 Uppsala, Sweden*, February 2000, Volume 7, Number 3, Pages 181-182,nature.com

29-Environmental Biotechnology. (Phytoextraction), Jan 31, 2011.

30-*Ritu Gupta and Giridhar U. Kulkarni,* Chemistry and Physics of Materials Unit and DST Unit on Nano science, Jawaharlal Nehru Centre for Advanced Scientific Research, Jakkur, Bangalore 560064, india. (A 'green' nanomaterial to remove organic impurities from wastewater), *issue of Nanotech Insights*, April 2011.

31- The-Compost-Gardener.com, (The Nitrogen Cycle - Nitrogen Fertilizer Nature's Way).

32-Biotechnology and Environment. (USE OF BIOTECHNOLOGY IN THE REMOVAL OF OIL AND GREASE DEPOSITS), Biotechnology 4U, copyright 2014.

33- Pro-Act Biotech. Oil-clean, 2012, proactbiotech.com

34- Deborah B.whitman., (Genetically modified food: harmful or helpful? Release April 2000, proquest.com

35- Sayer Ji. (Why GMO and Organic Cannot Co-Exist: Lateral Gene Transfer), Food Freedom.wordpress.com

36-FAO corporate document repository. Harvesting nature's Diversity, (Conservation and use of genetic resources).

37-National Human Genome Research Institute. (Cloning), genome .gov, *April 28, 2014.*

38- Advances in Immunology and AIDS Research. Sciencemag.org,

13 Jul 2001.

39- Herbert W. Virgin & Bruce D. Walker., (Immunology and the elusive AIDS vaccine), *Nature* 464, 224-231 (11 March 2010) | doi: 10.1038/nature08898.

40- DIAGNOSTIC METHODS IN VIROLOGY. Virology-online.com

41-Smith TF, World AD, Espy MJ, Marshall WF., (New developments in the diagnosis of viral diseases), PMID: 8345165(PubMed-indexed for MEDLINE).

42-Nature publishing group, R. W. *et al.* Evaluation of diagnostic tests: dengue. *Nature Reviews Microbiology* 8, S30–S37 (2010).

43-ANOVA medical center, (Stem cells in clinical practice).

44-EuroStemCell, Stem cell research updates from EU-funded projects, (Using time-lapse imagery to take a closer look at human embryonic stem cells).

45-Medical News Today (MNT), (Stem Cell Research News), 2014.

46-Rashed, Mortagy Dr., (Methods and advances in biotech), Trafford publishing, 2009.